Mentalizing Power and Powerlessness

Marie-Luise Althoff

Mentalizing Power and Powerlessness

Constructive and Destructive Use of Power in Psychotherapy

Springer

Marie-Luise Althoff
Bielefeld, Nordrhein-Westfalen, Germany

This book is a translation of the original German edition „Macht und Ohnmacht mentalisieren“ by Althoff, Marie-Luise, published by Springer-Verlag GmbH, DE in 2017. The translation was done with the help of artificial intelligence (machine translation by the service DeepL.com). A subsequent human revision was done primarily in terms of content, so that the book will read stylistically differently from a conventional translation. Springer Nature works continuously to further the development of tools for the production of books and on the related technologies to support the authors.

ISBN 978-3-662-66118-5 ISBN 978-3-662-66119-2 (eBook)
https://doi.org/10.1007/978-3-662-66119-2

This Springer imprint is published by the registered company Springer-Verlag GmbH, DE, part of Springer Nature.
The registered company address is: Heidelberger Platz 3, 14197 Berlin, Germany

Preface

Striving for power and the use of power often have negative connotations. People usually talk about their own powerlessness and the power of "those up there", and very rarely about their own striving for power. The everyday exercise or seizure of power happens unnoticed, secretly and is taboo. It seems necessary, in view of the phenomena of invisible power and also the increasing concentration of power and domination in our globalized society to confront oneself with one's own and other people's ideas of power.

"If you want to test a man's character, give him power", Abraham Lincoln allegedly said. Today it is usually countered that with power given not the true character becomes visible, but a new one. Possibly, the latter statement is only now true in our present time, in which character does not seem to be fixed but changeable, in which people work out multi-layered identities—against the background of modern individualization tendencies, in which concepts such as "crafting your biography", "patchwork identity", and "the flexible person" (Eickelpasch and Rademacher 2010) can be formulated.

Or can the so-called Stanford Prison Experiment (Zimbardo 1971) be taken as proof after all that the human nature is tending towards evil under certain circumstances, regardless of which era we happen to be in? The Stanford Prison Experiment, conducted by Philip Zimbardo with volunteers in the basement of the university's psychology department in California in the summer of 1971, was prematurely terminated in disaster after 6 days. The participants who had volunteered had been carefully selected and tested for mental averageness and health. And, with few exceptions, turned into power-obsessed guards and submissive, self-demeaning prisoners. Zimbardo assumes that when we get into a position of power, we are all thus in a new situation and can behave differently, thus form a different character. Zimbardo (2008) sharpened his thesis by suggesting that anyone can become good or bad under certain circumstances. What proportion of this must be attributed to the circumstances or the setting, and what proportion to the integrity or strength of character of the individual?

How can the individual maintain his integrity in the face of adverse circumstances? Nietzsche, for example, was concerned with overcoming powerlessness. He formulated a will to power: "Only where there is life, there is also will: not will to life, but—so I teach you—will to power" (Nietzsche 1980). Will to power, in his view, is demonstrated by a person's success in interpreting the world in the face of the powers of fate. This means, among other things, not to endure one's fate, but to want (better?) it. Wanting—according to Nietzsche—liberates from dependence and powerlessness. That is why the free man has "the greatest sense of power over himself". But if man wants to have certain experiences, then the question "Why me?" changes to "For what reason do I want to have this experience? What insights are associated with this experience?".

The experience of power and the exercise of power in relationships are examined in this book with regard to the effective factors of the internal framework of an individual, including ethics, morals, convictions about good togetherness, religious ideas, and the effective factors of the external framework, including human rights, laws, rights, institutions, professional codes, patient rights, psychotherapy guidelines, and the interactions of internal and external conditions. This makes it possible to highlight how the exercise of power and the overcoming of powerlessness can succeed in private and professional relationships, while at the same time incorporating the social context.

Imagine a person named Mr. Gutwille who is convinced that everything can be achieved or solved peacefully. What happens if someone puts something in front of Mr. Gutwille in a "surprise attack" that he does not like and does not want? For example, Mr. Gutwille and his wife may have recently purchased a townhouse in a new development area. One Saturday morning, he wakes up to loud shouting and hammering. He goes to the window. He sees that his neighbour has started to erect a fence (on his own property—so the neighbour is not breaking any law) with two other men. His wife is outraged, "He should have asked us. Go out and talk to him! By the way, I think the green of the fence is terrible". Both spouses experience it as a declaration of war coming from the neighbour. Mr. Gutwille does not think that he himself, for example, has failed to think about a fence and to contact the neighbour that he would now have to assert his claims. Instead, he defines himself as a victim of his aggressive neighbour and does not consider that he is thereby using undercover fighting techniques such as making no claims, remaining inconspicuous, being easy to care for, and that he is thereby acting with the aid of the power taboo, as a responder badmouthing the other and putting his own opinion above that of the other. I do not mean to say that these reactions of Mr. Gutwille are bad, so I do not want to judge them, but only to state that his reactions involve the use of a special power strategy by exploiting the power taboo. By the way, he is using a strategy that often involves self-harm and illness because it can become a battle of who surrenders first in the face of guilt.

The conscious decision to assert one's own will and interests is necessary and often even an ability essential for survival. I will examine why the ability to exercise power is nevertheless so hidden or disguised in large parts of our communication. In particular, the hiding of this ability also happens in psychotherapeutic relationships (Springer et al. 2005) although paradoxically the issue of dealing with power and thus the danger of abusing power are present in any therapy. The danger exists because of the asymmetry of the therapeutic relationship. Furthermore, there is the question of how power is exercised in psychotherapy on both sides.

In a first approximation, one could characterize the situation in such a way that a person seeking help with an unsolved problem, against which he feels powerless, comes to someone who offers knowledge and expertise, thus implicitly declaring that he feels powerful enough to be able to master the problem. This fact does not change even if therapy is understood as help for self-help. Conversely, psychotherapists are providers of a service that is also offered by colleagues. The person seeking help is therefore not dependent on the psychotherapist, can also switch to a colleague and thereby exercise power.

Suppose a patient, let's call her Ms. Spielviel, were with you for an initial consultation. The conversation goes well, you can imagine continuing to see her, and you offer her further appointments at the end. Now Ms. Spielviel smiles, "Yes, I felt good with you, but I have three more initial appointments with therapists I'd like to see as well". I am not suggesting that Ms. Spielviel's behaviour is bad or that she shouldn't do it this way, but that she is using her position of power and that you, as a therapist, might feel a sense of powerlessness in such a situation.

That power and the exercise of power in psychotherapy is a fundamentally inescapable issue on both sides and that should be indisputable. Yet psychotherapists are only just beginning to reflect on the constructive and destructive aspects of power. I understand this gap on the part of both psychotherapists and patients to be a mentalization deficit. Recently a supervisee asked me, when I spoke about the development of the destructive side of power in a psychotherapy she was conducting, whether there is also "good exercise of power".

The danger associated with a denial of power relations in psychotherapy is that destructive and abusive structures can be disguised and trivialized unnoticed, for example, by jointly shifting them to the outside, and then no longer be worked on, or that they can lead unnoticed to a malignant development in psychotherapy.

Psychotherapist Winsoft and patient Immerschwarz believe that they both suffer from the power exerted on them by the statutory health insurance. They are upset about it and cannot understand that the payer—in the person of the assessor—wants to know how long the therapy is likely to run and whether a good development is foreseeable. Both do not ask each other whether the other could not be more active and more helpful or more motivated and "whether the whole thing has already brought anything at all". Thus they exclude the power issue from their relationship. I don't mean to say that complaining together about the outside is bad, or that these latter questions are good in themselves. Perhaps each of us would even want to exclude such issues for the sake of convenience. In my opinion, Mr. Winsoft and Mr. Immerschwarz run the risk with an outsourcing of the power issues to the outside that their psychological general knowledge and their personal scope of action are expanded, for example, Mr. Immerschwarz experiences new dimensions in the therapeutic relationship such as being able to listen, empathize, authenticate, and be close—but that the dimensions of developing one's own assertiveness, one's own tactical and strategic thinking and behaviour are left out.

This book is about conscious and explicit use of power, is a plea for jointly negotiated power design and cultivation and for the acquisition of power competence on both sides. These themes are made explicit for the field of psychotherapy, but of course the potential applications are not limited to that (► Chap. 8). The case vignettes presented in ► Chaps. 5 and 6 are so altered from reality that identification of the respective patients and psychotherapists is no longer possible.

Among other things, you can expect answers to the following questions:

- Is it a bad thing to use power, to use influence to get your way?
- How can you learn to act powerfully?
- Where is the boundary between the constructive and destructive exercise of power?
- How can I enjoy constructive power games and get out of destructive power games?
- How can I overcome powerlessness?

- Do some situations require assertiveness and a certain distance and other situations rather closeness and credibility and persuasiveness?
- How can interventions and responses be evaluated in regard to their impact?
- How can we succeed in gaining an idea of the power of initiated consciousness processes and visions for the individual psychotherapeutic and private as well as social dimension?

Marie-Luise Althoff
Bielefeld, Nordrhein-Westfalen, Germany
Summer 2016

Acknowledgements

My heartfelt thanks go first to my wonderful family who encouraged and supported me during the manuscript writing phase. It was through everyone's patience that I was able to experience the strength to complete the book in the first place.

To all my friends, supervisees, and seminar participants who motivated me to turn to this subject and bring it to a conclusion, I thank you very much. To my patients and self-awareness participants, through whom I have been able to learn so much and who have been patient with me, I give special thanks.

The critical proofreading and the stimulating conversations with friends and relatives were a pleasure—many, many thanks for that!

I would like to express my sincere thanks to my office assistant, who has given me special support during this time and has graphically implemented the illustrations, for her loyalty and commitment.

I would like to express my sincere thanks to Monika Radecki from Springer-Verlag, who enthusiastically took up the subject of this book, always encouraged me and patiently accompanied me, and also to Sigrid Janke for the many encouraging words and the quick and uncomplicated help where it was needed.

I would like to express my deepest thanks to my editor Volker Drüke, who impressed me with his appreciative, careful, and at the same time competent-constructive suggestions for change and improvement. It was very helpful to be able to confide in his experience.

Lastly, I would like to extend my gratitude to the force of life itself that has guided me through this process.

Contents

About the Author

Marie-Luise Althoff
studied mathematics, psychology, and education; she is a psychoanalyst, lecturer, supervisor, and teaching therapist. She works in private practice in Bielefeld and teaches at several training institutes and universities. Areas of interest: secure Frame, mentalizing and mentalization-based treatment, and couples therapy. She is a founding member of the German-speaking Association MBT-DACH.

Introduction

Contents

M.-L. Althoff, *Mentalizing Power and Powerlessness*,
https://doi.org/10.1007/978-3-662-66119-2_1

1

Psychotherapists always work between the poles of power and powerlessness. It is striking that they are only just beginning to explicitly reflect this reality. In my opinion, one important reason is that many psychotherapists feel—to put it exaggerated—more like philanthropic idealists than egoistic materialists. Thus they usually declare that they do their work more for idealistic than for commercial motives. To that extent, then, it does not seem necessary to recognize or need to know the rules of the game of power. If one thought it was necessary, then one would have to justify one's own interest in the subject, perhaps even one's own striving for power, to oneself and to others. I think it makes sense to deal with the topic of "the exercise of power in psychotherapy" because our world today has changed into a society of "real existing neoliberalism" with a corresponding value system. By dealing with this value system I come to a positioning, which exercise of power should be called constructive and which destructive.

1.1 Psychotherapists and Their Self-concept

Although psychotherapists have always worked between the poles of power and powerlessness, it is only in recent times that systematic discussion of the topic has been initiated (Buchheim and Cierpka 2000) and demanded (Person 2003). The anthology "Power and Powerlessness" (Springer et al. 2005) stimulated the discussion.

All the contributions to be read there deal with the complexity of power and domination structures – both in the inner and in the outer reality – from a psychoanalytic perspective. On the one hand, psychotherapists are equally confronted in the treatment room with strange as well as their own concepts of power and powerlessness, with the temptation to act or enact them. However, they are challenged to deal with these ideas in an understanding rather than an acting way, and to make this understanding available to their patients. On the other hand, they are participants in public and professional politics. In order to actively participate in shaping these, they must continuously analyse their own fantasies of power and powerlessness.

Despite criticism of hierarchical power and training structures—formulated by Anna Freud, Michael Balint, Otto Kernberg and Johannes Cremerius, among others—little has changed at the level of training and further postgraduate training. This topic is also currently being reflected on in detail (Wiegand-Grefe and Schuhmacher 2006; Schmidbauer 2015; Thorwart 2015; Tibone and Schmieder-Dembek 2015).

Many psychotherapists have an unsettled relationship with this issue. I suspect that most psychotherapists feel more like philanthropic, altruistic idealists (φιλανθρωπ ος) than selfish, money-loving materialists (¢fil£rguron). Thus, most explain that they do their work more for idealistic than for commercial motives (Kernberg et al. 2005; Kämmerer and Funke 2004).

My own self-concept changed abruptly a few years ago when a good friend asked me why I would have so much patience and understanding for people with whom I have no family or friendship ties. Would I do it even if I didn't get paid for it? I was glad that the vast majority of were so close to my heart that I could say with an clear conscience that I would give my time even without money. I was a little uneasy about it, because if I didn't get money, I wouldn't be able to give so much of my lifetime. And what did I mean by "close to my heart"? Furthermore, I could think of a few people I would not have wanted to talk to without money. If I myself am now glad that I could and can use the word "few"—what is the danger? What was or is my motivation to offer psychotherapy to people in need? For me it is the good feeling of having been helpful, of being needed, of being trusted and appreciated. I became aware that this of course benefits others, but that it is *my* good feeling that makes the effort worthwhile or keeps me happy. As we know, altruism, unselfishness or charity, is as elusive as its counterpart, selfishness, self-love. Presumably they are two sides of the same coin.

In almost all social professions the so-called helper syndrome is discussed. This term was coined by Wolfgang Schmidbauer in 1977. He named the possible psychological problems in helping professions and summarized them under the term "helper syndrome". According to Schmidbauer, many people go into helping professions because they can unconsciously live out their own dependency needs there. Causes for this are located in the early childhood of the helper. In the end, it all boils down to the fact that the helper tries to be the ideal parent figure towards his clients, which the helper himself had fantasized in his childhood. This connection is often mentioned under the keyword "helping as defense". A side effect is that feelings and relationships with people who are not in need of help are often warded off or people are judged to be more in need of help than they are.

In one of my seminars on power, motivations for becoming a psychotherapist included spontaneously:

- Understanding and being able to understand
- sympathize/have pity
- Advocating for a better world
- Giving others the help you would have liked to have had yourself
- Help parents
- Alleviate trauma

Wanting to exercise power was discussed only secondarily by the participants—and "because it is the subject of the seminar".

It is now acknowledged that psychotherapies work (Meyer et al. 1991; Wampold 2001). If success is a given, then it might be unnecessary to reflect more closely on the subject of power, i.e. to try to recognise and apply the rules of the game of power. A disadvantage of such reflection could be that one would then have to question one's own self-image, perhaps even have to justify one's own hitherto unrecognised striving for power.

▶ Example

A very "poor" person, Mr. Niewasdabei, has made a second appointment with psychotherapist Vertrauensselig. He credibly asserts that he was again unable to arrive on time, this time the train did not come. At first Mr. Vertrauensselig thinks that Mr. Niewasdabei could have taken an earlier one just to be on the safe side. But when the "poor" man then reports that injustices always happen to him—he was already not a desired child, and then he was also supposed to be a girl—the psychotherapist can no longer protest when Mr. Niewasdabei says he is sorry, but he left his insurance card on the kitchen table. He was about to take it when the doorbell rang and the bailiff was at the door. He would certainly bring it with him next time, so the next appointment could already be arranged. Of course he knew that the insurance card was important, and he would surely get an appointment with the doctor tomorrow for the form (consultation report) that the therapist (!) needed. While a power specialist already thinks: "I'm not stupid, it's all lip service", Mr. Vertrauensselig still thinks: "Poor guy, I have to help him". He activates all his helpfulness, makes a new appointment and doesn't waste a thought on the fact that he is the powerless victim of a deception. ◀

1.2 Reasons for Rejecting Power

What makes psychotherapists, as well as other members of the helping professions, so easily forget or suppress their own interests, the awareness of their own power, their own striving for power or their own position of power? Is it the fear of not Measure up to the other person, which makes the psychotherapist take a defensive position, or is it, on the contrary, the fear of exploiting or abusing one's own power and superiority, ultimately the fear of one's own destructiveness, which is denied and, turned into the opposite, is reinterpreted as a helper position. This helper position, however, is then characterized by the powerlessness to influence the other. Then, often in return, one's own powerlessness must be denied out of fear of the destructiveness of the other person.

▶ Continuation of the Example

This circle of repression of power and powerlessness (on both sides!) could also have been set in motion in being with Mr. Niewasdabei. Without reading in the data from the insurance card, without having a consultation report and without bringing the signed therapy contract, not to mention the "forgotten" anamnesis questionnaire, Mr. Vertrauensselig starts to write the report to the expert in the open and trusting atmosphere and with the patient's assurance that the psychotherapist is the last one who can help. Power specialists would have been puzzled by the phrase "the last one". Of course, Mr. Niewasdabei is not aware of his power strategies. He has probably already fully settled into a victim identity and is suppressing the fact that he is making promises upon promises to the psychotherapist and not keeping them. He now pulls the psychotherapist deeper and deeper into his secret power strategies, which, however, he absolutely cannot recognize and experience as such. ◀

The question is how the phenomenon of Hidden takeover of power in helping professions, especially in our profession, can go unnoticed and how it can be countered. Why is it taboo to exercise power or to Exercise one's authority?

Psychotherapists are prepared to having to use their personality as the most important tool in their work. In this respect, one's own personality is constantly put to the test. There are personality constellations that are predestined for hidden or unconscious constellations of power and powerlessness. A prototypical example is the helper personality described by Schmidbauer (1977).

Childhood experiences that promote a taboo approach to power can be manifold, as the following examples show.

1.2.1 Excessive Search for Harmony

This can lead to denial of power scenarios. When children identify with the actions and behaviour of their parents and then to it accordingly themselves, they expect recognition and love in return. If the child feels that recognition is lacking, then the child may feel misunderstood and rejected by the parents. As a result, the longing for harmony, love and security can increase immeasurably and prevent conscious separation by assuming a position of power. There can be a tendency to boycott oneself – for the sake of recognition and love.

1.2.2 Dependence

A dependence on the guidance of others can lead to denial of power scenarios. Children initially experience their parents as all-knowing and all-powerful. They can usually detach themselves from this view by developing an increasingly stable ego ideal. If a person's ego ideal is not particularly strong, e.g. as a result of slights and devaluations, then he or she continues to orient himself or herself primarily to the parental guidelines anchored in the superego and does not perceive his or her own claims to power or is easily corrupted by the promises of others.

1.2.3 Unconscious Narcissistic Neediness

Unconscious narcissistic neediness can lead to denial of power scenarios. Children may come to believe that they are loved for their behavior or accomplishments, but not for themselves. In this case, a hidden unconscious narcissistic neediness may persist. People then seek validation of achievement as a way of satisfying their own hidden longing for affection, closeness, love and recognition. Since this succeeds only rudimentarily for brief moments and the environment usually does not understand this unconscious bartering, the striving for affection, closeness and love ultimately remains unfulfilled. The open expression of claims to power is not dared—for fear of then not being loved. Unconsciously, this sometimes leads to taking advantage of others.

1.2.4 Relations with People in Need of Help

The increased initiation of relationships with those in need of help can conceal the unconscious exercise of power claims. Children who are increasingly looking for love and recognition sometimes begin at some point to preferentially seek relationships with those in need of help, because they can then be sure of affection and gratitude, or can be "justifiably" angry in the absence of the same. As adults, they experience relationships with non-needy people as boring, superficial, unsatisfying, because they do not find themselves lovable or even valuable without the recognition of a helping activity. They themselves do not perceive how much they valorize themselves through the position of helper and thus exercise power. The effects of altruistic behavior out of defensiveness can determine the life of the affected person—up to the choice of profession and partner.

1.2.5 Indirect Aggression

Indirect aggression against non-needy people can be added from an (unconscious) feeling of powerlessness. Because of the experience or idea of not having been free in one's development in childhood, an unconscious aversive attitude towards normal social "free" relationships may arise. This aversion is often expressed in indirect aggression, such as defending the needs or rights of a third party. A feeling of powerlessness is experienced because non-needy people cannot be so easily "obliged" to show appreciation and gratitude.

As a consequence of these personality traits or a taboo handling of power, the psychotherapist can manifest that

- an ideology of the "good human" emerges,
- a personal altruistic value system is upheld,
- a high social conscience and sense of develops,
- Fear of their own unfulfilled neediness arise,
- fear of their own destructive develops,
- Fear of power and the exercise of power can be present,
- a high psychotherapeutic standard can arise,
- high pressure builds up due to the ideals conveyed in theories,
- a high pressure arises due to the social demands placed on psychotherapy,
- a tendency towards unconsciously disguised forms of exercising power intensifies (e.g. exercising power with reference to authority)
- high pressures due to incompatibility with the general trend of norms and values (► Sect. 1.1) develops.

It becomes clear that a tendency towards inhibition of aggression and rejection of open striving for power can already be deduced from the above-mentioned consequences. Now, of course, one could say that all would be well if all psychotherapists could throw overboard their open and latent misgivings about aggression and the striving for power.

Let us first see what happens further between Mr. Niewasdabei and the psychotherapist Mr. Vertrauensselig.

► Continuation of the Example

Presumably, the psychotherapist would not provide his own angry thoughts and feelings because he is not even aware of them (strong inhibition of aggression) or because he would not consider it purposeful (serving the patient).

Where would it lead if he were to show Mr. Niewasdabei his own power strategies in the process? "You put me off. You make promises to me and you don't keep them. You have overwhelmed yourself with your promises to me and instead of telling me, you drag me into your mess."

Perhaps Mr. Niewasdabei would say: "What do you want from me? You're the one who gave me new deadlines. And the fact that you started the report was your decision, wasn't it?" Then he would possibly leave furious for good, without having gained any insight about himself or the process so far. As an aside, the psychotherapist would also be angry by now "in the face of so much effrontery" and would have no insight into his own power strategies. Both would feel victimized. Then again, perhaps Mr. Niewasdabei would be depressed, saying, "Yeah, I'll never get it right." And would no longer come to the next agreed appointment and would also no longer be reachable by phone.

Of course, letting it go on like this, with delays, appointments not kept, provision fees not paid, therapy sessions not billable, is not an alternative.

Now what could be advised to Mr. Vertrauensselig if he wants to change the situation? He should think about how it got to this point in the first place, what his involvement is in bringing the situation about. He might remember, for example, that at the beginning, before he thought "what a poor man" Mr. Niewasdabei was, he was still quite aware that Mr. Niewasdabei had apologies, excuses, deceptions in store all the time. At the beginning he could have simply said, "Would it be possible for you to take an earlier train next time, just to be on the safe side?" I would now advise Mr. Vertrauensselig to

- ask himself what prevented him from asking this or a similar question whether he was e.g.—possibly not aware of himself—glad to have a specimen of the "needy" variety in front of him here and to be able to establish the hierarchy helper-needy, and
- write down a chronology of what happened in the form of: Who did what and when? ◄

If you find yourself in situations where you have agreed to something verbally or in writing in an atmosphere of trust, reliability and friendship or friendliness and with the affirmation of openness and helpfulness, and your counterpart does not keep his promises, puts you off, begs you, lies to you and drags you into chaos, then you are dealing with a power scenario.

Steps to Solve and Prevent a Destructive Power Scenario

- Through self-reflection or self-awareness, explore one's own involvement in this scenario, i.e. practice mentalizing the power scenario.
- Record measurable facts (who agreed to what and when, and what is the result?), and be sure to leave out any excuses, feelings, transference and countertransference considerations for the sake of clarity.

The presentation of the facts is important, because otherwise you might forget unpleasant details or immediately take the other person's side again. It would honor you if you would "not put things on the gold scale", "not make such a fuss", "not be so selfish" or "simply not be so stingy"—however, in such a situation you might then forget that you are thereby *unilaterally* restoring the good relationship. Compassion, helpfulness and understanding are not helpful to analyze the situation! Trust is only appropriate again when the actions of the other person speak for it. The more strongly one has developed traits of a helper personality, the more difficult it is to distance oneself from feelings and to relate completely to the facts. For there is a strong need to want to establish and maintain a good relationship, because one feels dependent on relationship.

Of course, I do not mean to say that compassion, helpfulness, understanding, transference and countertransference considerations are superfluous or even a hindrance. Likewise, inhibition of aggression per se and covert negotiation of the power issue are neither good nor bad. My question here is: How does one approach the issue of dealing with power while including one's own personality and resulting value system?

1.3 Hidden Value Change

Today's world is characterized by giving the development of the individual and his individual interests a high value—above those of the general public. Certainly, there is no such thing as *the* world of today. The trends, circumstances, experiences and fates are too different for that. All this requires an individual consideration, which, however, would go beyond the scope of this book. In this respect, I will only name a few formative currents of the time after the Second World War in Germany. As before, those born shortly after the Second World War are the decision-makers who are in power in politics, professional politics and business. They are those who still directly experienced the consequences of the war in the form of hunger, destruction and family trauma – caused by violence, flight or expulsion. The following birth cohorts from the mid-50s onwards grew into a time of repression and the incipient enjoyment of prosperity. The world was kept on tenterhooks by the threats of the Cold War, but at some point everyone calmed down with the fact that the superpowers were simultaneously keeping each other in check. For a long time it was not considered possible that a world war could threaten again at some point, at least that is what many say, for example, in view of the sudden uncertainty triggered by the Ukraine crisis in 2014.

In Germany, a system called the social market economy was established in the 1950s. Moral concepts were rather petty bourgeois, e.g. cleanliness, sense of duty, family orientation, religiosity, performance orientation. As virtues, diligence, accuracy, reliability, loyalty were at the top of the scale in school and work. Especially efficiency, readiness for action and striving for security were dominant values of this time. On the wave of Rock 'n' Roll a need of the children of the 1960s for pleasure, leisure, looseness came into all social spheres; especially the student movement and the sexual revolution angered and threatened the petty bourgeoisie of the

1960s. The climax was 1968, when the pressure on petty-bourgeois values became obvious, e.g. in the revolution at the universities, the women's movement, life in shared flats and wild marriages, Kinderläden (antiauthoritarian Kindergartens), the baggy look and long, open hair. Ideas were lasting peace and prosperity for all; there was an incipient environmental consciousness. The "oil crisis" of the early 1970s caused a brief irritation, but was then processed more under the ecological idea. Education should be accessible to all. Educational and advancement opportunities seemed to have little to do with origin and class. In this mood, Freud's idea of psychotherapy for the masses could also take root.

In West Germany, psychotherapy—initially limited to analytical and depth psychology-based psychotherapy—was introduced as a service financed by the health insurance system in 1967 (Rüger et al. 2015). Access to psychotherapeutic care was to be open to all; to this end, the concept of mental illness had to be brought into line with the Reichsversicherung's definition of illness. This has remained the case to this day, although with the issues of evidence-based and methodologically validated psychotherapy, new demands on the justification of psychotherapy come into play.

In the 1970s the declared goal was full employment, economic-political disputes were solved by consensus politics. The citizen could win: in 1975, for example, the construction of a nuclear power plant was blocked in Wyhl. The ecological movement formed out of the wild leftists and found a home with the founding of the Green Party. Socially, there were different currents. On the one hand the conservatives, who continued to follow the idea of performance and economic success, on the other hand the leftists, at whose extreme end the APO was formed, as well as those who turned to the inner life, who adhered to psychoanalysis, esotericism, psychology, free pedagogy or eastern wisdom. It was believed that peace had been permanently secured (despite the arms race of the two superpowers); the various currents (with the exception of the APO) were tolerated, sometimes smiling at each other generously. The basic consensus on a broad basis was free access to education and work for all. Psychotherapy financed by the health insurance system continued to gain strength. In 1987, behavioral psychotherapy entered the system (Rüger et al. 2015).

In 1989, the political situation changed relatively unexpectedly with the fall of the Iron Curtain, the unification of the two German states, the collapse of the socialist community of states. While the peaceful revolution was celebrated for many years, western capitalism was able to position itself as the winner and radicalise itself. With the help of transitional guidelines, the psychotherapeutic care structures of the New Federal States were transferred to care according to the (former West German) psychotherapy guidelines.

Capitalism seemed to be unleashed, the social market economy was invoked less frequently. The buzzword budgetary discipline was heard more and more frequently, and the spectre of the "unfinanceable welfare state" was able to make its appearance. The Maastricht Treaties tightened the disciplinary constraints on state budget management. It was made easy for the citizen to understand that the state had to save. At least that is what the running clocks of new debt showed quite strikingly and publicly.

At the same time, the Acts of war in Europe (Balkan crisis) caused a shaking of the people. The uncertainty had reached the population and favoured the change of values à la America in Europe, the change from the social market economy to neoliberalism. Why was there so little resistance to this? Perhaps it has mainly to do with the fact that the centre-left parties succumbed to the seductions of neoliberalism in rows. The Red-Green government under Schröder ("Comrade of the Bosses") said goodbye once and for all to working-class politics and a left-wing coalition. Even the trade unions got involved in speculation and had to collateralize losses with the members' strike funds. It was long overlooked how profits were maximised in the new system. While prosperity for all and private provision continued to be propagated and even the small investor was lured to the stock market, it became clear at the latest with the stock market crisis of 2001 that the fund companies and stock market goers had nothing but their own profit in mind. This was and could still be sold as a regrettable error, and many believed it, trusted their bank advisors and experienced in 2008 with the worldwide crisis triggered by Lehman Brothers, how all small investors, who had taken care of their private Retirement security on the advice of politicians, were ripped off mercilessly and the banks as system-relevant institutions were even supported by the state and at the same time made the biggest profits in this crisis. Meanwhile, we live in a time when the gap between rich and poor is widening, when more and more people need more than one job to have enough to live on, and at the same time many propagate that it is no longer about work performance but about finding ways to multiply one's passive income without working. This is favoured by the fact that income from work is taxed at a much higher rate—almost twice as high—as income from capital assets. The lower and the upper classes proclaim: Pretty stupid who works!

Resistance is now stirring across the board. There are forums opposing social cuts and uncontrolled privatization (e.g. of electricity, gas and water). While in the old EU states the left forces are strengthening again, the new EU states are succumbing to the seductions of neoliberalism. In parallel, we are experiencing military and terrorist threats; the Ukraine conflict is bringing back warnings of a world war for the first time; we are worried about the protection of our privacy.

Our current system shows a double face: on the one hand, it presents itself as cosmopolitan, dynamic and offering unprecedented opportunities and salaries for flexible, unattached, hungry, educated, loyal people; on the other hand, it is becoming a vision of terror for more and more people due to the transformation from appreciation to (economic) value added. Small and medium sized businesses, which used to be the pillar of the economy at about 90%, are increasingly losing their image, and on top of that are being disadvantaged in terms of lending as well as tax, while corporate giants achieve tax payments of practically 0% by employing highly paid shrewd financial advisors. And nobody seems to be able to do anything about it.

The fact that economic life is increasingly run according to the laws of war is evidenced by metaphors (e.g. the film "The Wolf of Wall Street", 2013); consultants from military circles are booming in the economy; psychotherapists are considered unsuitable as consultants in these circles. Psychoanalyst David Tuckett has written extensively on this area (Tuckett 2011) and can be consulted in more depth.

What has changed for the individual? In an emergency, everyone is supposed to fight for their own survival. The individual is given high importance; everyone is on his own.

Whereas in the past the legal and social state provided security and promised solidarity, today one is supposed to trust in security through capital accumulation; a capital accumulation which, ironically, is not within everyone's reach in view of the development of interest rates and investment opportunities. Care, humanity, solidarity are then at best lip service, which are however ridiculed in the case of emergency. Experiences of mortification and disparagement must be dealt with individually and in private. In the meantime, we understand that a change in values has taken hold almost unnoticed and insidiously. The people in the new federal states of Germany have felt this change much more blatantly.

At the very moment, we are being caught up directly and immediately by the war zones of the world, which seemed far away years ago—in the form of refugee flows. It is becoming tangible that in the near future there may no longer be any overall poor or rich countries, but only powerful, rich and powerless, poor strata in every country on earth.

Of course, these two positions, the social and the neoliberal, are not new, and I have deliberately presented the prevailing currents in a pointed way. As early as the sixteenth century, there was a theory—attributed to the prince Machiavelli—according to which, in order to achieve political power and economic influence, any means is justified—regardless of ethics and morality. Perhaps the difference is that so-called modern Machiavellianism is a nationwide phenomenon. Let's just look at the transformation of the term "authentic" so often cited in psychotherapy.

1.3.1 Authentic: Genuine and Honest or Credible and Convincing?

In the field of psychotherapy, the quality of authenticity has taken on an unimagined triumphant march. Statements such as "I want to be authentic in my reactions" or "Interventions only work if they are authentic" can be heard from psychotherapists of all practices. Competent, reliable, empathic, creative are desirable therapist traits, yet the pinnacle of efficacy, the sum of all virtues, seems to be associated with achieving authenticity. But what does that mean? Is it not the case that a psychotherapist at the end of their training, or at different stages of their professional life, would each describe different responses of their own as authentic? Stern (Stern et al. 2012), for example, mentions that he is so socialized by his analytic training that it is authentic for him to remain silent for minutes at a time in psychotherapy sessions. Is this intervention then, just because it is authentic, appropriate or effective?

We generally understand authentic behaviour to mean

- to act openly and honestly,
- to show yourself the way you feel,
- not to pretend,
- nothing to hide.

Authenticity and genuineness of personality are highly valued. This attribution derives from a value system in which the psychological view of the world is highly significant. Certainly, these values are invaluable important in family and friendships, especially in love relationships. But can this attitude be transferred to the professional world? Psychology, education, and the social sciences reinforce that our world would be more humane and healthy if we were all authentic in the sense of “open” and “honest” and “genuine.” The variables of authenticity and truthfulness have been central to all forms of self-awareness since Rogers.

But can one really recommend participants in self-awareness groups and group encounters to always and without exception show themselves with their sensitivities and feelings? Power experts would absolutely deny this, even call it “suicidal”. They would never expose themselves to such a risk without carefully examining the situation. At most, they would advise others to show themselves quite openly in order to be able to better assess the other person.

But isn’t authenticity something that career and business advisors also advise professional politicians and officials to do? No, not in the sense just described; they advise to be authentic at all costs, in the sense of “appearing credible” and “being convincing”! The goal is then

- being able to convince,
- give the impression that one is convinced of one’s own method,
- to be suggestive,
- come across as sympathetic.

So the goal would not be to tell the truth, but to achieve that the listeners of a Christmas or New Year’s speech, an advertising event, a lecture, a psychotherapy session believe you, find you likeable, feel comfortable and act and go by according to what they have heard or experienced. When the listener gets the impression that the speaker is convinced of his message, finds him humanly agreeable, trust and suggestibility grow. The speaker himself does not have to believe what he is saying. The speaker is interested in “getting his message across” in order to achieve a higher goal. For example, a psychotherapist may say, “Of course there is a good chance that this psychotherapy will help you get well!” because early questioning could radically diminish the patient’s hope of recovery. A career politician can formulate a campaign promise that will help him win. And he can thereby buy the time to prove himself in politics. If he then finds a way to distract from the unkept campaign promise, he has the power to expand his position and can gain even more power and influence.

But isn’t this attitude immoral? Doesn’t one then lie to the face of others? Doesn’t one then use elaborate deceptions? The question is whether it is an alternative to tell the patient from the beginning that his condition can also worsen through psychotherapy, and to risk that this fear then possibly leads exactly to that result. Can the politician forego unrealistic campaign promises and then possibly not get a chance at parole, simply because he will not be elected? Should a manager of a corporation risk speaking authentically-honestly about the board of directors’ preliminary plans for massive staff reductions and thus risk that this announcement will cause the stock price to plummet and “his head to roll”?

Those who answer these questions in the affirmative are more likely to fail in asserting their goals and will also be encouraged in their self-conviction "The main thing is that I am honest" by power experts. However, this is not because they would have done it in the same way, but because they are then sure not to be attacked or overtaken by this colleague. They are happy to be able to control and easily lead this person. The power experts themselves just have to appear as if everything is sincere and give as good explanations as possible for the discrepancies between promises and actions. In this respect, in our modern world, one is at a massive disadvantage in many areas of professional life if one behaves authentically-genuine instead of authentically-credible.

Perhaps you have noticed how during my argumentation you have gradually recognized in yourself that you also sometimes behave authentically-genuinely-honestly and sometimes authentically-credibly-convincingly. When you hear the word authentic or use it yourself, the meaning will vary depending on the context. And it is worthwhile to assess your counterpart as to which meaning is currently meant.

▶ Example

Mrs. Ehrlich was outraged: Health insurance payments had fallen sharply. With starting a family, building a house and opening a practice, existential fears came to the fore. Of course, it was not only Mrs. Ehrlich who was affected and beside herself. Colleagues in all parts of the country joined forces. Mrs. Ehrlich found that in some parts of the country there were even already well networked structures and precise ideas about a nationwide union. The founding of a new professional association took place, and Ms. Ehrlich was even elected to the federal board, then to the representative assembly of her Professional representation and as a deputy delegate to the representative assembly nationwide, due to her commitment, which resulted from her great concern and her ideas of justice. In these bodies, the factual questions suddenly stood seemingly on an equal footing with the questions of preserving one's own positions, defending the conquests of one's own specialist group and one's own professional association. Skillful tactics and negotiation were implicit in every agenda. One fellow board member was sympathetic to her, and she discussed much with him. One day it became apparent that this colleague had taken advantage of the position within the group to excel and move up in another organization with discussion results that others had worked out. Initially stunned and disappointed, but then thoroughly intrigued and with a realistic assessment of her own strategic abilities, Ms. Ehrlich decided against further involvement in professional politics because, as she said, "it doesn't suit me." ◀

Even if one is not involved in professional politics or on a similar stage, I consider a concrete confrontation with the topic of the exercise of power in psychotherapy to be overdue in view of the change in values described, because patients also have to come to terms with the change in values. In doing so, they need our support for their daily struggles in family, circle of friends, kindergarten, school, studies and the world of work, and we therefore cannot or should not form an enclave in our practice. It is not tragic that power is often exercised not or secretly. It only becomes tragic when—figuratively speaking—the Trojan horse is pushed into one's town and the inscription "I am weak" or "I want to sell you something very special at a cheap price" obscures the true content. Where would it lead us if we withdrew in our daily practice almost exclusively into the niche of preserving the old values and morally rejected the inclusion of the new values or left the confrontation with them to others?

Of course, we are not a homogeneous group of the "eternal yesterdays"! Since we as a group certainly do not always and everywhere, nor do each of us want to withdraw or retreat to the same extent into this niche, I would like to illustrate my basic thoughts on the power strategies that different people use, pointedly and with the help of a metaphor. Imagine a nation in which there are two groups, the altruists and the highest-performers (I would like to avoid using the word "Gutmensch" here, which took 2nd place in the election of the un-word of the Year 2011).

▪▪ Altruists

The do-gooders have certain norms and values. You can recognize them by the fact that they know and can quote do-gooders like Rousseau, Marx and Freud. They would say of themselves that their heart is in the right place. They are generous, bona fide, believe in the good in people; they are very altruistic and politically correct. Their moral sense is strong and can go to the point of being opinionated. Values they hold are humanity, moral courage, solidarity, social justice, socialism, idealism, pacifism, feminism, anti-racism. They are represented in the ecology and alternative movement, have a positive attitude towards esotericism and New Age, are critical of the media and strive for an anti-discriminatory attitude. They are committed to community, to the welfare state, to redistribution from rich to poor in the sense of equalizing justice, to the provision of public services as a task of the state, to health care and education freely accessible to all, to solidarity with developing countries. They are opposed to neo-liberalism and the excesses of globalisation and more often express the wish for stronger state control. They feel closer to the working population than to big business and the holders of exposed positions of power. Authority is quickly suspect to them, their threshold for attack is low, they feel morally superior and consider their goals ethically superior. They are often seen by others as ridiculous, pushy and arrogant, as "social romantics", "minded terrorists" and "unworldly idealists".

▪▪ Highest-performer

The Highest-performers, on the other hand, see themselves as materialists, monetarists, Calvinists, and thus justify their individual striving for profit. If everyone would take care of himself and be egoistic, everything would go well automatically, "as if by an invisible hand", in freedom and self-regulation. They advocate free competition and against state regulation and communist egalitarianism, for the development of the individual's capacity in competition. In their view, neoliberal capitalism has emerged as the only functioning system, the winner. Unions hinder success and are ultimately to blame for unemployment because companies have to go abroad. Globalization without regulation would lead to prosperity and peace for all. The typical Highest-performer is performance-oriented, disciplined, structured, organized, commercially thinking, strategic, tactical, confident in negotiations, assertive, self-confident, loyal, with an intact family and lives according to the motto “Everything must pay off”.

1.4 Old and New Value Systems in Competition with Each Other

Is one system obsolete and the other that of the future? No, certainly not; I merely want to sensitize you to observe yourself more or less agreeing sometimes with one side, sometimes with the other.

The altruists are of course also not free of intentions and desires and also come under pressure. However, they then behave more like stressed parents, they nag, complain, don’t get their way, are offended or make accusations. They don’t set consequences because they don’t want to disturb the peace or spoil the mood. Do the children then do what is asked?

The prototype of the exclusively cold manager who would sell his grandmother, who in case of doubt would even rationalize himself away, is a horror scenario at the other end: constantly in work and stress, afraid for his job, threatened by loneliness and in pressure to conform due to the obligation to double-talk in terms of lip service to social compatibility. A modern Machiavellian, for example, cannot say publicly that a production must be moved abroad because it might cost him his job immediately if it disadvantages his company. He can hardly talk about his strategies and has to take high risks and perhaps “unlearns” to be able to open himself to love relationships at all.

Altruist versus highest-performer—whose power strategies are sensible and forward-looking, especially in the field of psychotherapy? Or is there a third way that helps us out of the moral dilemma? Of course there will be new developments, and each of us can contribute to them. In this book I point out individual ways and solutions. We as psychotherapists, when we are in the status of freelance or self-employed, have comparatively large degrees of freedom. Nevertheless, we have an obligation to take an interest in the tensions that arise for our (usually working) patients from the everyday tussle for power. Otherwise, we tend to profit from the social upheavals without helping our patients to cope with them, or possibly even increase their pressure. We therefore have to deal with power strategies on two levels (▶ Chap. 4):

- with the socially prevailing power strategies in order to better understand and be helpful to our patients,
- with the socially prevailing power strategies, in order to recognize which strategies we ourselves (unconsciously) use, and to decide which ones we want to use and which ones we consider harmful.

To stay in the picture once again: Which way of life brings which advantages?

Advantages of the Lifestyle of the highest-Performers

- Openly striving for power can be done in harmony with oneself, does not have to be denied.
- Motivation to reach a top position can be lived openly.
- Permission to be authentic-credible is compatible with goals.
- Wanting to use power of feelings and empathy is compatible with values.
- Wanting to learn self-control, -regulation is compatible with goals.
- If long breath is strategically required, the other can be left out.
- If laws of the soul are to be used, they can be exploited.
- When valorization of an individual's performance is to be done, one has no qualms.
- If someone can tell a good story, that art can be recognized.
- If someone wants to use suggestion, this can be welcomed.
- When numbers, facts, results are critical, you don't let feelings get in the way.

Advantages of the Altruist's Way of Life

- When social and human motives prevail, one knows oneself accepted by others.
- When competition is shied away from, one assures oneself of the goodwill of the other party.
- If partnership is to be lived, one can dedicate oneself to common goals.
- If it is a love relationship, emotional closeness can be experienced.
- If a community project is desired, common good can be realized.
- If the counterpart also argues morally, it is possible to come to an understanding about morality.
- If sharing emotions and motivations is desired, one can explore and share one's inner life with others.
- If dramatizing sensitivities is part of it, you meet like-minded people.
- If solidarity is desired, one can feel strong in community.
- When emotional surprise attacks are used to overpower the opponent, immediate passion and liveliness are lived.
- If the real level is the most important thing, there is no need to invent a story.

In this comparison, rather an ideal-typical discussion is sketched out to illustrate that one prefers different behaviours depending on context and goals. Value system and strategies must fit the situation and oneself. Only then can the individual feel and live his integrity. It is postulated that one always uses power strategies in social interaction. The strategies chosen then differ depending on the value system and situationally depending on the intended goals and the nature of the relationship. I assume that every relationship can be located somewhere on the continuum from absolute love relationship to absolute service relationship.

In psychotherapy, each therapeutic relationship is certainly to be located on a different point of this continuum, for neither are psychotherapeutic relationships purely love relationships (understood here as emotional relationships) nor purely service relationships. The determination depends, among other things, on the following questions: Does a basis of security and trust exist in the concrete psychotherapy? What is the attitude of my counterpart? Are the parties involved aware that closeness is important for psychotherapy, but that economic interests also play a role? Can I trust enough to develop my attitude as I speak, or do I have to be clear about what I want to say beforehand? Can I assess my counterpart? What indications of credibility and trustworthiness do I have? What consequences and ways of dealing with them are recommended? What could I use to build up pressure if necessary? When has the relationship matured enough and is closeness possible so that I can show authenticity in the sense of openness and honesty?

In order to be able to be clear about all these aspects in the therapeutic relationship, to know when one strategy is appropriate and when the other is appropriate and, at best, to be able to exchange ideas about them, one needs a lot of social competence.

I understand power competence as part of social competence.

Wherever one lives and works, it will never be possible to completely avoid proceeding strategically to one's own advantage in order not to be at a disadvantage or to be able to achieve certain goals. Cost-benefit analyses are helpful here. It is more or less a matter of professional survival. In friendly, helping relationships or in love relationships, however, the use of these strategies is harmful. Those who are only concerned with their own advantage will quickly disappoint and lose family, patients and friends. Emotional closeness comes from trust, tolerance, openness and honesty, from giving the other person insight into one's own motives and intentions. These closeness variables do not change with new social reference or value systems; they are universal.

The following chapter will focus on how power and the desire for power can be mentalized and how power competence can be acquired.

References

Buchheim P, Cierpka M (Hrsg) (2000) Macht und Abhängigkeit. Lindauer Texte. Springer, Berlin Heidelberg

Kämmerer A, Funke J (2004) Seelenlandschaften. Streifzüge durch die Psychologie. 98 persönliche Positionen. Vandenhoeck & Ruprecht, Göttingen

Kernberg OF, Dulz B, Eckert J (2005) WIR: Psychotherapeuten über sich und ihren "unmöglichen" Beruf. Schattauer, Stuttgart

Meyer AE, Richter R, Grawe K, von der Schulenburg J-M, Schulte B (1991) Forschungsgutachten zu Fragen eines Psychotherapeutengesetzes. Bundesgesundheitsministerium, Bonn

Person ES (2003) Feeling strong. How power issues affect our ability to direct our own lives. Harper Collins, London

Rüger U, Dahm A, Dieckmann M, Neher M (2015) Faber/Haarstrick. Kommentar Psychotherapie-Richtlinien, 10. Aufl. Urban & Fischer, München

Schmidbauer W (1977) Die hilflosen Helfer. Über die seelische Problematik der helfenden Berufe. Rowohlt, Reinbek bei Hamburg

Schmidbauer W (2015) Kann eine (Lehr-)Analyse ungültig sein? Forum Psychoanal 31:53–68
Springer A, Gerlach A, Schlösser A-M (eds) (2005) Macht und Ohnmacht. Psychosozial-Verlag, Gießen
Stern D et al (2012) Veränderungsprozesse. Psychosozial-Verlag, Gießen
Thorwart J (2015) Zur Prävention von Grenzverletzungen in der psychoanalytischen Ausbildung. Forum Psychoanal 31:35–51
Tibone G, Schmieder-Dembek B (2015) Abstinenz und Abstinenzverletzungen in der psychoanalytischen Ausbildung. Forum Psychoanal 31:17–34
Tuckett D (2011) Minding the markets. Palgrave Macmillan, Basingstoke
Wampold BE (2001) The great psychotherapy debate: Model, methods, and findings. Lawrence Erlbaum Associates, New York
Wiegand-Grefe S, Schuhmacher M (2006) Strukturelle Gewalt in der psychoanalytischen Ausbildung. Psychosozial-Verlag, Gießen

The Development of the Mentalization Ability

Contents

M.-L. Althoff, *Mentalizing Power and Powerlessness*,
https://doi.org/10.1007/978-3-662-66119-2_2

The starting point of this chapter is the question of how one can mentalize power and the desire for power and thus acquire the basis for power competence. The ability to reflect on oneself and others as beings with mental states is referred to as mentalization. First of all, it is presented how mentalization ability develops in children under conducive conditions, at what age children can think and act strategically, and what dangers parents and caregivers should keep in mind. The fact that different mentalization abilities can have serious effects on flexibility and competence in dealing with power is illustrated by way of example. A high mentalization ability seems to be advantageous. In this respect, the topic of stimulating mentalization presents itself as an important psychotherapy task for the patient and often also for the therapist. Different patients (as well as therapists) need different ways of stimulating mentalization.

2.1 What is Mentalization?

The English term "mentalization", coined by Peter Fonagy and Mary Target, is derived from the adjective "mental" or the noun "mind" (Latin *mens*, relating to the mind). It is used, for example, to refer to "mental illness" and "mental condition". In German, the term cannot be translated literally; the English "mental" means spiritual, mental, psychic and soul at the same time. In this respect, the English term "mentalization" has been translated/transferred into German as "Mentalisierung" (mentalization), since there is no German term that encompasses the comprehensive meaning of the English "mentalization".

Mentalizing means the ability to interpret the behaviour of other people or one's own behaviour by accepting mental processes or states (cf. Fonagy et al. 2004a). In doing so, reference is made not only to the behaviour of the other person, but to one's own ideas and fantasies about his or her inner world, such as thoughts, beliefs, desires, intentions and attitudes that produce this behaviour.

> Mentalizing means to assume what is going on in the mental system of another person based on his or her behavior. The intention and the attempts to grasp and explain one's own experience and behavior can also be understood as mentalization.

Imagine you are in a café watching a couple engaged in a loud exchange of words. You cannot understand the words because they are speaking a foreign language. You observe violent gesticulation and serious expressions. What are you thinking and feeling? You may suspect that the two are arguing and have different positions. So far, the assumption can first be deduced from the observable behavior, the signs. But it may be that you automatically suspect the inner states of the two people and develop feelings yourself that you think might correspond to their feelings. It could be that you think that the couple is in a crisis and that you are experiencing feelings of sadness, fear and that memories of self-experienced conflict situations arise. Then, from one second to the next, both partners smile; they stand up, take each other in their arms and walk out of the café hand in hand. You are left behind confused, and if you are lucky, a person who knows the language enlightens you that the two disputants did not have a partnership dispute or even a crisis, but a dispute about what mentalizing actually means. Mentalizing is omnipresent in everyday life and usually occurs automatically, just as you immediately and without conscious intention imagined what was going on in the café. You can always be more or less "right" with these ideas.

To be able to mentalize requires a basic implicit understanding of the nature of the mental. Essential to this is the knowledge that reality is only represented in our minds or psyches, that thoughts and ideas simply approximate the real world. The ability to mentalize is largely unconscious or preconscious. It is a cognitive and emotional performance that gives meaning to one's own behavior and that of others. Learning to mentalize is part of self and ego development and enables meaning making, understanding, thinking as probationary trial, and reflection as a tool of impulse control and affect regulation. Under normal developmental circumstances, the ability to mentalize develops in its essential components by the end of the 4th year of life and differentiates through increasingly extensive experiences until adolescence. Maturation depends on life circumstances, relationship and attachment experiences and affective exchange with the first, but also all later attachment figures.

It is essential for the significance of the concept of mentalization for psychotherapy that the ability to mentalize can, under certain conditions, still mature in later years of life. This is an important prerequisite for the improvement of perceptual, regulatory and communication skills.

Unfortunately, especially under physical or psychological pressure, the ability to mentalize is quickly reduced to a greater or lesser degree. We recognize this by the fact that

- we don't feel so balanced anymore,
- we can't act so prudently anymore,
- we see the other(s) more negatively or even as enemies,
- we restrain ourselves, even though we know that action now could have an unfavorable effect.

This means that just when we could use the skill the most, we often have it least available, e.g. when

- there's a dispute or misunderstanding,
- we are unexpectedly confronted with crisis situations,
- strong conflicts of interest emerge abruptly,
- intense feelings, e.g. disappointment, distrust, feeling cheated, arise,
- wants, needs not met in relationships important to us,
- severe traumatisation has occurred or is to be dealt with,
- in psychotherapies, intense feelings of guilt or shame,
- we are under intense pressure of conscience,
- we're afraid to exercise power,
- we feel helpless and powerless.

To it: In psychotherapy, the goal of shared mentalizing is to learn to distance oneself from impulsive, destructive, and/or self-destructive behavior in these kinds of pressure situations by beginning (initially together and consciously) to reflect rather than act automatically, e.g., to feel the disappointment or fear, to notice it, to observe it, and not to act "headlessly" right away. Allen et al. (2011) talk about hitting the 'pause button'. This is helpful in giving oneself time and being able to regain power over oneself and the situation. This applies equally to the psychotherapist and the patient.

For example, a psychotherapist might say, "I realize I haven't quite figured it out yet. I'd like to think about it for a minute. Maybe we could do that together." Or he might say to the patient, "Maybe you could manage to hit the pause button for a moment in these kinds of situations at home." Or a patient might say, "I don't understand what you just said, what are you talking about?"

2.2 How Does the Ability to Mentalize Develop?

Mentalizing as a cognitive and emotional performance does not develop by itself with brain development, along a maturation line, but is acquired in relationship, i.e., the person recognizes himself through the other. Infants are thought to be able to feel well-being or discomfort prenatally, triggered by certain events. However, they have no awareness that they themselves are "happy" or "angry" or "anxious" and by what or by which person these sensations were triggered. The research group around Fonagy considers the development of the ability to distinguish emotional states and to assign them to categories to be very important. This ability makes it possible to recognize one's own emotional states as such, and it forms the basis for being able to attribute mental states to other people in the further course of development.

2.2.1 Early Affective Mirroring (up to About 9 Months of Age)

Fonagy and Target refer to György Gergely and John Watson's (1996, 1999) model of affect mirroring to explain how infants develop the ability to perceive and differentiate affects. Gergely and Watson describe the process of conscious affect perception on the part of the infant, which occurs in interaction with his caregivers. If this process is successful, it also provides a basis for the development of the ability to regulate affect. Fonagy and his working group agree with Gergely and Watson (1996, 1999) that babies still perceive their emotions and the physical feelings that accompany them in an undifferentiated, unreflective and correspondingly vague manner (they speak of "primary awareness"). It is further postulated that infants become more aware of their own states first through the reaction of the caregiver to their emotional expressions, namely through a response of the caregiver that corresponds to the baby's emotional expression. Or, to put it another way, the baby finds itself in the other; parents or caregivers, in turn, without thinking about it (it is assumed to be biologically inherent behavior), respond to the baby's expressions of emotion in specific ways. They communicate with their baby in the so-called motherese or baby-talk. This language is characterized by a heightened pitch, much repetition, a simple vocabulary, and exaggerated emotion expression in response to the baby's emotion expression. They mark their mirroring emotion expression as exaggerated and as a mixture of different affects (including soothing parts, if necessary), so that it becomes possible for the baby to recognize that the caregiver is responding to him (referential anchoring on the part of the baby), that it is not just the caregiver's expression (referential decoupling on the part of the infant), and that *his* state is being played with (awareness on the part of the infant). With a successful phase of affect mirroring up to the age of about 9 months, the foundations of mentalization ability, namely affect perception and differentiation, are established. In these first months the infant develops along the at best sufficiently good contingent and congruent mirroring a feeling of life, which is described as **contingency experience.** Thereafter, an increasingly complex world view develops in dealing with external reality.

2.2.2 Developmental Steps of the Further Mentalization Ability

Targeted Mode (From About 9 Months to 1.5 Years)

The goal-targeted mode is also called teleological mode. The child can grasp its own and other people's actions from observation and interpret them as goal-directed. Own trial-and-error behaviour is directed towards a goal. It can perceive authorship. However, it cannot yet recognise underlying causes such as motives, intentions, desires, and it can easily be deceived.

During this time, object permanence (Piaget) develops, in which the child realizes that an object or person continues to exist when it is outside its own field of perception. Parallel to this, the so-called eight-month fear or stranger anxiety also occurs, because the child can now distinguish which persons are familiar to him and which are strange and scary. It reacts to faces that are unfamiliar to it in a dismissive or tearful manner.

In psychoanalysis, object constancy (object understood here as person) is formulated as an achievement of the age of about 18 months. What is meant is that the child has developed a constant attachment to the primary caregivers and can maintain a relationship relatively independent of need satisfaction. A child who has acquired object constancy has a concept of mother and father even when they are out of sight and hearing, even if this state is relatively unsatisfactory to the child at the moment. Care and concern continue to be felt even in temporary absence. It can be assumed that this feeling of closeness to the caregiver also implies continuing to have a sense of one's own existence, one's own self, and not feeling abandoned. At the same time, successfully getting through such periods of absence is also the basis for the child's growing experience of courage and confidence in being able and allowed to lead his or her own life.

Is there already social competence at this age, especially power competence?

Researchers at the University of Portsmouth led by Vasudevi Reddy (2008) studied more than 50 infants and toddlers with their parents using tests and skilled questioning and came to some astonishing conclusions regarding infantile deception. The earliest form of purposeful deception in humans, they said, was tactical crying. For the first six months of life, babies cry elementally, unrestrained, with force and without "ulterior motives." From the age of about half a year, the study found, children feign crying and, a little later, laughter to attract their parents' attention. In addition to hunger and discomfort as driving forces, there is soon the intention to want to be close to the caregiver. The child already knows how to direct its environment quite well, because it knows exactly the effect of tears: men as well as women break out in a sweat. Generally, they try to stop the crying by nurturing, caring and caressing the child. Then the child has achieved its goal. Two months later, children seem to have a (still crude, of course) idea of "right" and "wrong" and can cover up "forbidden" or mislead their parents with diversionary tactics.

Parents see through this more or less well. These early forms of conducting can certainly be understood as preliminary forms of social competence, more precisely leadership competence or power competence.

▶ Example

If you let a ball roll just past a goal from a short distance several times and quietly say, "Oh, no," the 9- or 10-month-old baby crawls up, pushes the ball into the goal and smiles at you in satisfaction. It doesn't yet see through the fact that you could just as easily have let the ball roll into the goal yourself. ◀

- **Psychic Equivalence (From Approx. 1.5 to 4 Years)**

At this stage of the development of mentalization, the child cannot yet distinguish between thoughts and external (for sure). Inner states such as thoughts, ideas, fantasies, wishes and fears trigger similar sensations and feelings as real events and are not distinguished from them. In psychic equivalence mode, the infant thus experiences the internal world as identical to the external world. One's own thoughts are perceived as real and identical to the thoughts of others. Everything is concrete for the child, concretistic from an adult point of view. The child cannot yet understand that thinking and desiring are representations and interpretations of the environment, not reality itself. As a result, one's own affects or fantasies, which exist only in the imagination, are potentially attributed effects in reality and are thus experienced as fearful.

Parents ideally deal with their child's experience in two ways: They take the child's inner state seriously, e.g. make the child understand that they can perceive and understand his fear, but provide another perspective by checking the reality, thus also showing that they are not frightened.

▶ Example

If the child thinks in the evening that there is a crocodile under the bed, then this idea seems so real and threatening that it no longer dares to get out of bed. When it has summoned the father, the father then turns on the light, he acknowledges the child's fear and reassures the child by not showing fear himself and initiates that they both look under the bed, the child agrees with the father's explanations. This does not mean that the fear does not reappear when the light is off and the father has left the room again. ◀

▪ Parallel: Pretend Mode (From Approx. 1.5 to 4 Years)

The pretend mode is understood to be a state in which reality is suspended in the child's experience, quasi nullified. Inner and outer reality are decoupled. In this mode, the child can play absorbedly without fearing that the play will have real consequences. In this way, the child can represent his inner states and create representations externally (without being aware of it). As a result, the thoughts and desires and impulses that occur in fantasy remain harmless, or are fantasized to have been mastered with the help of fantasy. This mode has also often been called magical thinking. A famous example is Freuds grandson's Cotton reel game described by him (Freud 1920): his 1½-year-old grandson had repeatedly thrown a wooden spool wrapped in string over the edge of his crib so that the spool rolled under the bed, only to pull it out again with great delight. He commented on the disappearance of the spool with a sound meaning "gone," and on its reappearance with a joyful "there." Freud interpreted this game as a staging of the mother's departure and return, as a discovery of overcoming suffered powerlessness through playful activity, that is, coping with the experience of separation by shifting it to an object that can be brought under control.

The role of the parents is to understand the play action as a production. Through their comments on the play actions, they can verbally mirror the child's inner states by playing along, i.e. marking the child's actions and emotional expressions. Ideally, destructive fantasies and desires are also worked through in play, whereby the child needs a co-playing adult or an older child at his side for this, in order to be able to remain firm in the conviction that an idea is only an idea, which does not directly affect reality.

► Example

For example, if the child plays father-shooting, along too realistically in the shooting game can cause the child's fears to burst in abruptly. If such a game is forbidden, the child may think that the desire to play shooting is already evil. In both cases the child would be in danger of tipping over into equivalence mode, i.e. in one case thinking that the father would now be dead, in the other case thinking himself to be evil because he wanted to play an evil game. ◄

These play experiences organize and mediate between the modes of mental functioning of the equivalence mode and the pretend mode, so that the child can more and more confidently maintain his mentalizing stance and experiment in a trial-and-error manner.

How does social competence or power competence show at this age?

Even as two-year-olds—at the height of their own conception of greatness—children master tactical tricks, although the maneuvers are still easy to see through or can be misguided. If the expected effect does not occur, the child shows his anger and defiance very violently in an attempt to achieve his goals. However, thinking about the inner life of others is only possible to a limited extent, so that children as young as two years old sometimes use throwing away their pacifier or destroying their own toys as punishment for their parents (cf. Kohlberg's stage model in ► Sect. 2.4).

This is where parents with their patience and mediating skills are needed. If children at this age are not limited in an understanding and gentle way, the claims to power and leadership that are blatantly shown at this age, which are also definitely underlined with the use of physical means such as hitting, pushing, for example, on the playground or in kindergarten, can remain unmodified and possibly lead to major problems at school. Play as a medium enables control and modification (pretend mode), and the playfulness of the caregivers prevents the overly harsh intrusion of reality (equivalence mode).

Furthermore, in the age range from 1½ to 4 years, the toddler's range of experience expands enormously. The motor skills, the cognitive development, the emotional experiences require an expansion of social skills. Thus, with the formation of empathy and empathy, it also becomes possible to move from egocentrism to the inclusion of the desires, ideas, and intentions of others. It is still difficult for the toddler to defer his own needs, but beginnings of altruistic cession can be observed. Siblings with each other who feel unobserved by adults can still be very cruel to each other and far from being kind to their brother or sweet to their sister, but they know full well that this is what the parents expect of them. In the presence of the parents they do not show the aggressive behaviour if possible and try to deceive the parents into believing that they are "nice" to the other. If the parents come into the room unexpectedly, the person who was beaten seconds before can be stroked—a shrug of the shoulders is also not unusual, accompanied by the statement: "I don't know what he/she has either". Even suggestions that are declared to be "for the other person" still relatively transparently pursue one's own interests. For example, the two year older child may say, "Mommy, we'll put Daniel to bed first, he's always so tired in the evening, and then you can play with me, the game he doesn't like." The significance of sibling constellations and especially sibling rivalry is a significant topic (cf. Leman 2004; König 2008; Sohni 2011) that requires further investigation.

■ Reflexive Mode (Approx. from 4 to 5 Years of Age)

The reflexive mode integrates the previously coexisting and alternately used equivalence and pretend modes. Reflection on one's own self and on the presumed inner lives of others becomes possible. Different perspectives are acknowledged, and false beliefs are included in self and others. The child explores what the actions of others mean, based on this they can learn to determine their own mental experiences and recognise them as meaningful (Fonagy 2003). The concept of mentalization is essentially based on the idea of shared experience (Fonagy and Target 2006): the ability to reflect from the age of 4 becomes possible when the child has been able to experience that his or her mental states are reflected by the caregivers.

> » The child now perceives the connection between inner and outer reality, while at the same time acknowledging that they differ in significant aspects and need neither fall into one (equivalence mode) nor be dissociated from each other (pretend mode). (Fonagy and Target 1998, p. 32; note in parentheses: the author)

How does social competence or power competence show at this age?

At this age, reaction-formations (related to siblings) result at best in a caring attitude. The social conscience is more pronounced and mature. Primary school children know exactly what is unfair and are nevertheless selfish:

▶ Example

While exchanging Pokémon cards, it was clear to the little boy that he was about to get ripped off. Instead of offering him at least the desired (not at all rare) card and one other card for his five cards, his friend had only offered him the longed-for card if he would add one more of his cards on top of it, and one that he didn't actually want to give away. Just the one and then put the valuable card on top of it! On the other hand, he didn't know if he could still buy the card he longed for, and he didn't want to wait anymore. What should he do? Refuse? To him that would have been no great matter. At least he wouldn't have given his mean friend anything either, but the friendship was in question now anyway. He wanted the one card so badly, though! He agreed, even though he knew it was an unfair trade.

It looked similar on the other side. The friend also knew that his offer was unfair, but he also knew how badly his friend wanted the card and couldn't resist the temptation to get as much out of it as possible – even if it meant running the risk of not only upsetting his friend, but also losing him. ◀

But are we really evolving, or are the same strategies simply executed more covertly and thus more perfectly in adulthood? It is possible that the division offers of primary school pupils are not in line with the ideas of parents, teachers and educators, but they are not so far away from the adult trade agreements that go by supply and demand or power and influence.

▶ Example

For example, the right to access to clean water was recognised as a human right by the United Nations General Assembly on 28 July 2010. However, as became known in 2014, this does not prevent a company like Nestlé from pumping the water directly from under the feet of the population in Africa, for example, and then exporting it. Human dignity, decency and responsibility for society as a whole are called for in vain. ◀

Although children of primary school age already have a fairly strong sense of moral justice and fairness, this does not mean that what they themselves have morally identified, felt and verbally expressed as right is also what is expressed in their actions. Studies have shown that strategic action against one's better judgment is not particularly pronounced in children up to the age of 13.

Researchers led by Tania Singer of the Max Planck Institute for Human Cognitive and Brain Sciences in Leipzig (Steinbeis et al. 2012) postulate that this has to do with the development of their brains. The dorsolateral prefrontal cortex—a region in the frontal brain responsible for impulse control—only matures gradually. It fits with these findings that children have astonishing problems putting abstract knowledge about equitable distribution into practice.

Singer and her colleagues had 146 schoolchildren between the ages of 6 and 13 play two classic games from behavioral research: the ultimatum game and the dictator game. In the dictator game, the dictator can make an offer regardless of what his counterpart thinks or feels—and the other person must accept it. Giving more than necessary here without need is benevolence and generosity. In the ultimatum game, on the other hand, players must factor in the other person's reaction. If one becomes too impudent, the other can punish this behaviour—and both receive nothing. In this respect, those who give more are not acting altruistically, but are trying to minimise their own risks.

As expected, the offers from the children playing Dictator were almost universally outrageous. In the Ultimatum game, by contrast, the older a child was, the higher the offers. Surprisingly, the researchers said, younger children between the ages of 6 and 9 in particular were much more likely to accept unfair offers in the game. However, if they were asked about it theoretically, without a concrete gift beckoning, they did not want to let the other person get away with such impudence.

In the study, it did not matter how intelligent or empathic a child was, how well he or she could empathize with others, or whether he or she was prone to risky behavior. The decisive factor in behaviour was willpower. There is thus evidence that gaining power over oneself in the form of impulse and regulatory control is an important goal for the upbringing and education of children.

2.2.3 Development up to Adolescence

A continuous improvement in the ability to reflect is measurable with the expansion of the background of experience into early adulthood. For Fonagy et al. (2004b), adolescent crises should not be understood—as is often the case—as normal inner chaos or drive breakthroughs, but as a consequence of earlier developmental deficits that are only now becoming apparent. Due to the developmental demands of detachment from parents, adaptation to the peer group and the impending demands and uncertainties in studies and work, it is easy for earlier conflicts to be reactivated. Traumatic stresses from childhood are then enacted (in teleological mode or equivalence mode) or denied by escape from reality (in pretend mode).

Although neurofunctional changes in the brain are structured by sex hormones, adolescents also have increased activity of subcortical structures (limbic system), while the maturation of prefrontal control areas is delayed (prefrontal cortex: planning of behavior, reflection and emotion control). This then leads to a specific imbalance, as the more mature limbic system initially gains the upper hand over the not yet mature control system. And this connection also explains increased risk-taking behaviour and a lack of reflective ability and behavioural control.

But this does not mean that adolescents are no longer in control, it just means that the demands on their regulatory and impulse control skills are increased (Konrad et al. 2013). The reflective competence that adolescents acquired in childhood is crucial to their ability to cope with the demands of puberty and adolescence. And it is possible that good mentalization skills make the prefrontal cortex grow faster!

2.3 At What Point Can Children Become Strategic in Social Interaction?

The results and considerations reported in the last section suggest that although deceptive manoeuvres are already possible in infancy and toddlerhood, they are not brought about deliberately and willfully "with ulterior motives" or "an awareness of deception" as a moral category, but are motivated by needs such as hunger, discomfort or closeness. Babies do not yet design cognitive strategies in the strict sense:

> Children up to about 3 years of age are naïve realists, they unquestioningly hold the way the world appears to them to be true and accessible to all, they do not yet understand that their beliefs about facts are only assumptions that can meet or miss the real facts. (Bischof-Köhler 2011, p. 330)

Only from about 4–5 years of age, with the understanding of the connection between inner and outer reality, the integration of equivalence and pretend modes and thus mentalizing in the reflexive mode are possible.

Thus, in the interplay of brain maturation on the one hand and social relational and attachment experience and guidance on the other, mental development moves from a mental reality in which mental states are not mapped as representations to an increasingly complex view of the inner world characterized by the ability to presuppose thoughts, feelings in others and in oneself, and also to recognize that there is a connection between these and the external world.

It is possible—especially with the guidance of older children or adults—from the age of 5 or 6, in principle, for the benefit of a desired goal achievement or long-term perspective realization

- to be able to lose, for example, to get the respect of a friend,
- to be able to share, for example, not to go empty-handed the next time,
- putting needs aside in order to be accepted in a community, for example,
- understand irony, for example, not to get angry at the other person,
- understanding jokes, for example, to develop more understanding of the inner life of others,
- to punish/ignore someone by not paying attention, e.g. to express one's disapproval,
- to recognise when one is being treated unfairly in order to be able to take action against it, for example,
- to discuss which strategy is better (without knowing the word strategy), e.g. to be able to achieve something with others that is not possible alone.

These abilities are, of course, still limited by the horizon of experience and the cognitive possibilities of this age group. For example, Piaget has shown that children in the concrete-operational phase cannot yet consider as many variables simultaneously as children from the age of 12 or 13 who have reached the formal-operational phase. In this respect, strategic abilities are still limited in their complexity. With increasing age and the possibilities of abstract thinking (the formal-operational phase), strategies can also be designed with medium-term or long-term goals in mind.

Imitation learning is of great importance in social interaction (Bandura 1976). Essential for the fact that behaviour is imitated or the observed behavioural strategies are used are the expectations that someone associates with the imitation. Referring to Bandura (1979), who highlighted three levels of expectations, I would like to name these levels in their importance as motivational stimuli for strategic behaviour of children and adults.

2.3.1 Expected Results

The behaviour of a model is preferably imitated if one expects pleasant consequences or thinks that unpleasant consequences can be avoided. Thus, expected behavioral consequences become an incentive for behavior.

▶ Example

Andi's friend reports that he has been learning vocabulary for half an hour every day and has now written a good grade. Andi envies his friend that he no longer has to be afraid of not being promoted and now hopes to be able to achieve this by doing the same and also learning vocabulary every day. The expectation of results (transfer), which he expects, is therefore an incentive for him to learn. ◀

2.3.2 Competence Expectation (Also Self-efficacy Experience)

When a learner observes a behaviour in a model, the observer must also have confidence in himself to perform this behaviour in order to actually want to imitate it or to be able to demonstrate it. The learner thus makes a subjective assessment of his abilities, which he needs to imitate the behaviour. This is called the phenomenon of competence expectation. A person is most likely to perform a behaviour if his own expectation of competence is relatively high.

▶ Example

If Maria is asked at a ski jumping event if she would like to jump off the hill, she will only do so if she thinks she can handle it. ◀

2.3.3 Expectation of Self-affirmation (Also Self-regulation)

People judge their behaviour according to certain subjective criteria and can affirm themselves. From this follows the expectation of a favourable self-assessment when adopting a behaviour to be imitated, which then in turn leads to satisfaction and well-being.

▶ **Example**

Marcel, who rejects cheating on moral grounds, will hardly be persuaded to imitate this behaviour by observing a fellow pupil showing his cheat sheet, even if there is the prospect of external reinforcement, such as a better grade. ◀

2.4 What Dangers Should Caregivers Be Aware of?

Normally, parents, teachers, educators and guardians, i.e. all caregivers, want children to behave in a thoughtful and purposeful way, possibly even strategically. At the same time, child education and training usually emphasize that behavior should also be socially acceptable and not exclusively selfishly oriented. This means that caregivers—certainly for different motives—always convey that in addition to the expectations someone develops for themselves, the effects on others should be considered. How can this influence on the part of the caregivers in the various developmental phases of mentalization idealtypically look like?

▪ Phase of the Teleological World View

Early forms of cheating should be taken humorously, but you should smile and show that you have seen through the situation, and not always be directed. This is difficult for children when they realize that they do not get what they want. And incidentally, of course, it's also difficult for adults who are still predominantly in that mode. There is no sense of injustice at this level. One should strengthen the expectations of results by making it clear to the child what advantages there are in taking the others into account, e.g. letting them play along.

▪ Equivalence Mode Phase

In this phase, it is important to take children's fear seriously, but it is also important not to let fear infect and direct oneself. At the same time, one should carefully address the fact that fear of punishment also has its justification, for example, if one simply wants to take something without it being one's own.

▪ Phase of the Pretend Mode

Children should be able to experiment with trickery and theatre in a playful way, but not so intemperately that reality moves out of the world. Children must also be able to try out lies, but it is important that they experience where the limit of trying out lies and where real consequences threaten or what dad or mom no longer find funny.

These attitudes and measures should help the children to realistically assess their expectations of competence and their own experience of self-efficacy and to learn to tolerate deficits. It is helpful to have self-affirmation and self-regulation exemplified by the adult caregivers.

If a child has acquired good mentalizing skills over the first four years of life, there is nothing to worry about as a teacher or educator or as a parent; children can understand and practice strategies to control their impulses—by learning from the model—and thus succeed later as adults.

▶ Example

Walter Mischel from Columbia University in New York was already able to prove that there is a connection between impulse control in childhood and success in later life. In the 1960s, he put a marshmallow in front of four-year-old children. If they didn't touch it until another adult came into the room, they would get two, they were told. Some couldn't stand that for half a minute; they immediately went for the candy. Some children, however, started singing, turned around or distracted themselves in some other way and were able to resist the sweet temptation for up to 20 min.

Mischel tracked what became of these children for more than 40 years. The result: those who were able to distract themselves from the immediate reward were more successful in their professional and private lives decades later. Saving money, dieting, giving up smoking, completing a lengthy education—all these things came easier to them. ◀

■ Reflective Mode Phase

From the phase of the reflective mode onwards, it is possible to assume that children have a conscience to which appeals can be made. In this context, it is of particular interest to keep in mind as a caregiver which stage of moral development a child or adolescent may have reached or has concretely reached.

Lawrence Kohlberg (1974) is known to have postulated six stages of moral development—based on Piaget's stage model of cognitive development. It is worth briefly recalling the research method: The subjects were presented with the so-called Heinz dilemma (in different variants), which was formulated in its basic form as follows. The husband Heinz is faced with a moral dilemma: His wife is terminally ill, and only a drug, which is however far too expensive for him, could help her. Is he allowed to steal to save his wife, or must he let her die? Kohlberg made it clear that it is not a subject's **solution that** is crucial, but the way in which a solution is argued for. He highlighted three phases with two subcategories.

The Three Phases of Moral Development (According to Kohlberg)

Preconventional morality stage (up to 9 years and some adolescents and adults, e.g. offenders).

1. moral principle: opportunism and goal: avoidance of punishment
2. moral principle: egoism and goal: self-interest

Stage of **conventional morality** (majority of adolescents and adults)

3. Moral principle: Social norms and goal: Social esteem
4. Moral principle: Legal norms and goal: Acting in accordance with social order

Stage of **post-conventional morality** (few adults after age 20).

5. moral principle: utilitarianism and goal: greatest possible benefit for society
6. moral principle: universalism and goal: independent reflection and consideration of ethical principles.

According to Kohlberg, a person must make progress in three areas to move from one level of moral consciousness to another:

1. His social perspective must broaden: from an egocentric perspective to a realization of the claims of other people in the community.
2. His moral self-determination must increase: he must be able to question and justify moral norms.
3. The justification of the rules of his actions must gradually change: from a purely egocentric justification according to desire or dislike to an increasingly abstract, post-conventional justification of norms.

Lies, deceit and deception must be understood in their nuances, and people can develop morally-ethically according to role models and fateful events. There was a critique of Kohlberg's model in the 1980s (Gilligan 1983). Carol Gilligan, for example, points out what she perceives as the basic problem of science, androcentrism, and thus struck a sensitive nerve in the 1980s. According to Kohlberg, women are much less likely to reach the highest level of morality he defines (level 6), which he attributes to **deficits** in women's socialization. Gilligan, however, thinks that Kohlberg sets the specifically masculine as the norm and universally valid. In a study she puts forward the thesis that there are two equally valid forms of moral judgement. In her opinion, the form of morality specific to men is oriented towards abstract principles (**fairness, rules and rights as a guideline**), whereas the form specific to women is oriented towards social principles (**care, compassion and concern for others**). These two forms involve **conflicting responsibilities**, neither of which, in my view, need necessarily be typically male or female. It is also possible that moral judgments differ intra-individually, depending on whether they concern heart or business relationships.

2.5 What Is Part of the Social Competence of an Adult?

With the formation of conscience and moral development, social competence also develops.

> » Social competence refers to the ability and willingness to work together with others in a goal-oriented manner, to grasp their interests and social situations, to deal with them rationally and responsibly and to communicate with them, as well as to help shape the world of work and life. (Definition of the German Qualifications Framework for Lifelong Learning, ► www.dgr.de)

Social competence ("social skills" or "soft skills") thus refers to the individual attitudes and abilities that help to combine one's own goals with the interests and values of a group and also to influence the behaviour and attitudes of this group. The aspect of **social competence that** is sometimes equated with "social skills" is **social intelligence** as the "ability to understand others and to behave appropriately and intelligently towards them" (Sowarka 1995, p. 365).

In the literature, "soft skills" are often referred to as the abilities and skills which, in addition to social competence in the narrower sense, also include inclinations, interests and personality traits such as resilience and frustration tolerance. "Soft" is used because these abilities and skills cannot be measured as reliably via tests as "hard skills", i.e. professional competence or typical occupational qualifications.

In different milieus of a cultural group and even more so in different cultural groups, the expectations that are placed on an individual in a particular situation can be very far apart. Thus, in the face of comparable situational demands, different behaviours can be assessed as competent. This means that a person who is considered socially competent within a certain milieu may be assessed as socially incompetent within another milieu, in a similar situation. In this respect, there cannot be, for example, a definition of behaviours that can be regarded as socially competent in social situations (cf. Stangl 2001; Hinsch and Pfingsten 2007).

Building on the skills of affect perception, affect differentiation, and self-object differentiation, as well as self-coherence, identity security, and cognitive maturity, social competence is composed of the following skills, among others:

Skills of Social Competence

- Ability to work in a team
- Willingness to cooperate
- Communication skills
- Conflict Management
- Intercultural competence
- Empathy
- Critical faculties
- Oral and written expression skills
- Ability to consider the views and interests of others
- Engagement
- Self-motivation
- Leadership

I would like to take a closer look at the ability to lead. One sometimes encounters the idea that the ability to lead is something given, something that cannot be learned, or something that is quasi-inherent only in certain charismatic personalities. On the whole, however, the idea has prevailed today that leadership competence can also be acquired like a craft by learning and training certain skills.

These skills include general context-independent skills and, more recently, increasingly also very specifically defined skills that companies and organizations consider necessary for their own leadership positions. Leadership competence cannot be defined exhaustively in general terms from the perspective of an organisation or company, but must be defined separately for that particular company and hierarchical level as the sum of company-specific behavioural expectations. It would go too far here to go into detail about specific leadership capabilities formulated by specific companies and organizations. Examples of special skills are detailed expectations of what is to be understood by result orientation or willingness to take risks, which are then formulated very differently in concrete terms depending on the industry and hierarchical level.

In the following, I refer to general descriptions of "soft skills for the leader", which belong to social competence and focus on the ability to lead, influence and represent others. For example, Julia Kuhlmann and Julia Schmidt write:

> In order to climb the career ladder, you need not only the professional know-how and many years of experience of a future manager, but also the appropriate soft skills. No matter which industry you prefer: social competence will get you ahead everywhere. (► www.staufenbiel.ch)

In general, the ability to lead is understood as being able to lead, motivate and represent employees. Social skills then subordinate themselves to this goal. Leading, motivating and representing employees requires skills:

- **Prerequisite**

Perseverance, discipline, organizational skills

- **Communication Skills**

This includes being able to discuss and negotiate objectively. For example, the manager is expected to be able to give presentations in an appealing manner and in an appropriate tone and to conduct discussions with customers and employees. Fluency and confidence are considered essential for a manager to be able to represent the interests of the company. In contact, a confident and sovereign attitude should secure the respect and recognition of business partners and staff.

- **Judgment**

Managers should be able to assess the performance of employees and also accept their criticism. It is considered indispensable to be able to accept feedback and to use it for oneself, because this makes it possible to become aware of one's own strengths and weaknesses and to be able to work on them. In addition, an exchange with employees is considered an important step towards employee satisfaction.

- **Diplomacy**

The art of diplomacy is usually considered particularly important for managers. With the ability to deal with conflict and the effort to maintain perspective even in deadlocked situations, as well as with tolerance, fairness and a high degree of empathy, managers should succeed in conducting disputes, clarifying misunderstandings and working out compromises.

- **Engagement**

Extensive commitment characterizes the activity of managers, e.g. to engage, for example, in employee motivation through variation of tasks, and through targeted use of praise and criticism. It is assumed that the work attitude of the manager also has an effect on employee motivation in the short or long term. Leading by example is considered an absolutely effective motivational tool.

- **Delegate**

"As a boss, you should be able to take on certain tasks. These include, for example: agreeing on goals, delegating and controlling tasks, promoting and developing employees, giving feedback, motivating and informing", writes Sabine Olschner (▶ www.staufenbiel.ch). In addition qualifying enterprise-internal and external seminars are offered. The exchange with trainers or experienced managers should also help to familiarise oneself with the different areas of responsibility.

- **Empathy**

In addition to leadership tools in the narrower sense, social skills are also considered important, e.g. responding to and listening to employees. It is assumed that the better a boss knows his employees, the better he can use them for the various tasks. Confident knowledge of human nature and good powers of observation are just as essential as empathy, self-confidence and assertiveness.

- **Further Education**

Today, employees can hardly get into management positions without participating in further training and seminars on personality development. Participants learn how they should react in certain situations. In addition to theoretical tools, experienced trainers also provide simple "learning by doing."

- **Find Your Own Style**

Aspiring managers are taught about the different leadership styles. For example, there are seminars that are advertised with the following words: "You will learn that you can lead your employees in a strongly authoritarian manner by setting them narrow limits. If, on the other hand, you choose a democratic style as a leader, you will give your team the freedom to decide many things for themselves. If you decide on a partnership style of leadership, you will meet your employees at eye level," writes Sabine Olschner (▶ www.staufenbiel.ch).

In summary, the skills that belong to general social competence also belong to leadership competence to a large extent; however, they differ in their target orientation, which generally goes more in the direction of teamwork and cooperation and, with regard to leadership competence, is centered on the ability to lead. Special skills are important when dealing with employees:

- be able to provide information
- be able to motivate
- be able to represent
- be able to direct
- able to agree on goals
- able to delegate and control tasks
- enable employees to develop and grow
- be able to give feedback

Otherwise, the skills of social competence apply, i.e. perseverance, discipline, organisational talent, communication skills, rhetorical skills, diplomacy, conflict management, tolerance, fairness, empathy, commitment, initiative, secure knowledge of human nature, good powers of observation, self-confidence, assertiveness, authenticity, choice of the appropriate leadership style.

In both private and professional contexts, the development of social-emotional competencies, including leadership competencies, is a multi-layered development that is always accompanied by, or can be described as, the development of mentalizing ability in this area. When it comes to the topics of power and powerlessness, "mentalizing under pressure" is often required in social relationships, whether in the family, at school, at work or in psychotherapy. Something has to be said quickly, countered, decided, defended against, and possibly when feelings of competition, grudging, envy, jealousy, greed, avarice, winning, losing, fear, shame and guilt resonate. In the following chapters, you as the reader can develop your ability to mentalize under pressure on the topic of power and powerlessness by exploring the dimensions of mentalizing on the topic (initially without pressure) as you read the text and, stimulated by it, beyond. The ultimate goal is to be able to encourage patients for whom this seems necessary and meaningful in the area of power and powerlessness to mentalize in this way.

2.6 Is Power Competence Automatically Included?

Social competence and thus also leadership competence include power competence, because competences are used, for example, to achieve something oneself, to influence others, to communicate with others in order to achieve something, to tackle resistance. However, having or wanting power is often only present as an unspoken, implicit motivation. It seems naturally important to achieve one's own goals without jeopardizing the relationship. There may be a fear of losing the relationship by explicitly claiming power. In this respect, claims to power are often concealed and tabooed from oneself and others.

It can be useful to realize that you can only change your behavior if you know and control your emotions. In this respect it makes sense to be aware of one's own will to power and also to know what one's intentions are. There is nothing reprehensible about emotionally directing one's fellow man if one is aware of one's own emotional integrity and motivation. Moreover, one influences a situation in any case, it is only a question in which direction. If you go into a meeting grumpy and grumbling, you will earn the displeasure of your colleagues. If, on the other hand, you appear smiling and friendly, your positive attitude will create a good mood, make you feel better and you will probably even be more successful in getting your ideas accepted (cf. Goleman 2008).

In order not to fall for systematic and continuous manipulation, it is important to be able to impute the will to power to other people and at the same time not to succumb to one's own vanity or a desire to belong. Zimbardo (2007, p. 250) writes that "a powerful influence to transform human behavior, a force that makes people cross the line between good and evil, arises from the fundamental need to be 'in' rather than 'out'".

Everyone behaves strategically! It is only a question of the goal that someone wants to achieve.

Consciously open	Conscious and covert	Unconscious and implicit
Heart relations	Business relations	"Altruistic" helping
Community	Competition	Ideology
Model	Fraudulent intent	Consensus
Noble intentions	Self-protection	Sense of life
	Taking advantage	

It is therefore a matter of expanding mentalization to develop, post-mature, explicate, expose and de-taboo the subject of power and also of powerlessness in psychotherapy.

2.7 When is Power Mentalized and How Can Power Competence Be Acquired?

You basically mentalize the issues of power and powerlessness throughout your life, especially in threshold situations.

Initially, issues of power and powerlessness are experienced and mastered in the family, often in living together with parents and siblings. In the process, fundamental (unconscious) convictions about who one is, what place one should occupy, and how powerful and self-determined, but also how powerless and helpless one (unconsciously) fantasizes oneself to be, emerge.

With these convictions and feelings and the experience of oneself, one usually comes to a day care centre or kindergarten and experiences that quite different ideas and laws may apply there and that other people, children as well as educators, do not necessarily behave according to one's own expectations. These experiences can have a direct impact on one's own experience of power or powerlessness. For example, a child might feel powerful in the family and experience rather small and helpless in the kindergarten and might then develop a fear of the kindergarten situation.

Similarly, when entering school and in the further course of school, it will first be the case that it is not predictable what experiences of power and dominance or powerlessness and inferiority await the child. In contrast to the kindergarten situation, however, the demands increase continuously, because less and less protection can be given by the parents, the responsibility for the performance area should gradually and continuously pass over to the child's own responsibility, because the teachers—at the latest from the transition to secondary school—no longer automatically take care of the emotional well-being of a pupil, because the peers become more and more important and exclusions can cause quite violent shocks to the self-confidence and the view of oneself.

With the start of a course of study or vocational training, as well as later entry into the profession, come great demands. Depending on how the separation from the parents has succeeded and how strong and powerful one feels, this step succeeds more or less well. But it can also be the beginning of a story of suffering. This is often connected with an (unconscious) experience of feeling trapped in powerlessness.

Feeling powerful or powerless and wondering why that is, usually and at the latest, comes up when you enter into partnerships. Some feel (unconsciously) so powerless that they do not even dare to take this step. If it seems reasonably good for one, one dares the step into marriage.

Then most plan or have a child or children. If you thought until now that you had your life under control, that you actually felt quite powerful, you will find out when living together with children that you are led to limits, limits of your own power, your own control and self-satisfaction. In short, you experience helplessness, being at the mercy of others and powerlessness, or you have to repress and out a lot in order to be able to stay in a feeling of power.

Some go into psychotherapy at this point, if they didn't need help before, and then it becomes absolutely important to look at the issues of power and powerlessness together over the course of life, so that patients can rediscover the meaningfulness of their own lives and learn to distinguish between what has to be accepted and what can be changed.

Usually, at some point, the view widens for each of us to deal with areas that go beyond the normal family and individual framework, e.g. how to deal with illness, trauma, violence, accidents, death, chaos, society, religion, war, world peace. Themes of power, empowerment, domination as well as powerlessness, submission and sadism always play a role in reflection and coping.

Now a few examples of problems in which mentalization on the themes of power and powerlessness could be stimulated in psychotherapy:

2.7.1 Mentalisation to Break a Taboo

A 19-year-old young man registers for psychotherapy because in the last year before graduating from high school he is increasingly lacking motivation and is saddened and feels powerless and as if he is foggy. He claims to have had a happy childhood, to have experienced no major setbacks himself or in the family, such as accidents, illnesses, separations. He does not take drugs, does not drink alcohol. In fact, he found that he always been a good student, at least he had never been at risk. At the word "at risk," I inwardly bristle and think, "Where could the danger be now?" Further interaction reveals that he has plans to go to college, but, he says, as it stands now, he won't be able to start the study. I ask what comes to his mind when he hears the term "start". He says that what comes to his mind is that one starts a service, a military service or war service.

In many sessions of joint work it emerges that for him starting studies means something like going out into life and having to prove himself. Unconsciously, he seems to associate this with great danger. When I ask if anyone in the family has ever been harmed, he says, "My mother's brother, when he started into military service." He is visibly moved as he tells the story of his uncle and his mother's grief, which is not talked about.

One (of many) meanings that his phase of pathological disturbance had was that a taboo had formed in the family as a result of the traumatic event (uncle's accident during military service): **You must not become strong, because then ...** This taboo had combined with his own age-appropriate fears and anxieties on the threshold of his studies. He was able to finish this "then" hesitantly. "Then I'll fail, then I'll come to death like my uncle because I'm too sure of my powers, then my mother won't be able to cope and will sit there powerless and unable to do anything."

In another case, a 37-year-old patient with a psychosomatic disorder reported, among other things, that she was very successful in her job and had now been offered a position. This could be the crowning glory of her career. I asked her if she was sure that at the age of 37 there was still a more to come. Spontaneously she says, as if rushed: "Then I would have surpassed my father. That scares me. That can't happen. How could it with my illness?"

As it went on, it turned out that—objectively speaking—it could happen relatively easily that she could still reach a higher position (than her father). It became clear to her that her physical symptoms acted as a brake. We were able to consider where the sentence **You must not become better than ... Dad** came from, but above all what a professional position had to do with "being better".

2.7.2 Mentalization in Order to Build up Mentalization Skills in General

A man comes to couples therapy with his wife. Among many other issues, he reproaches her for being so unbearably hard on the children that she is also inconsiderate towards him, so that he no longer dares to express his wishes. These complaints reach a temporary climax in the sentence **I can't deal with ...** my wife's Self-aggrandisement.

It was difficult for him to reflect on his own desires, why he had originally been attracted to his wife, and why this collusion had occurred in their relationship. It was also difficult to fathom what this might have had to do with his primary family as well, that he had gone into the powerless position like this.

In another case, a 15-year-old adolescent whose parents had separated in a highly contentious way reported in the anamnestic interview that her boyfriend had left her. He had been unfaithful, unreliable and violent, but she still could not let go of him. Since then she has been cutting herself, constantly writing him messages and lurking around him. She always thought he was the one and she would do anything for him, and she wondered how she could convince him. She can't stand being so powerless. She's like, **"I can't get over this."**

It was necessary to clarify many areas together in small steps in a long-term therapy, to differentiate affects and to work on self-object differentiation.

2.7.3 Mentalization to Overcome Powerlessness

A 52-year-old patient who experienced severe trauma in his childhood tells that he is being bullied again at work. Both the boss and the foreman were constantly demanding more work or more speed from him. He thinks that he tries everything, but never gets any peace. **Again and again Spokes are put in my wheel** …

In the psychotherapy it became very clear that (unconsciously) whenever he was in expectation of calm, he perceived everything that then appeared as a difficulty as if it related directly to him, as if the others were only behaving in such a way to hit or hurt him. He was willing to explore reality to find out what he could do himself to better separate himself internally and externally.

Another patient, a mother of five children, says that she always thought that when the children were all over ten-years old, they would be out of the woods. But now she realizes that there is always something that makes it even more difficult. She says that she so exposed. **Why Does it Always Have to Be Difficult for Me … ?**

We were able to work on her unconscious pathogenic belief that had existed since early childhood ("If I serve others, then I have a right to be there and be part of the family"). With the reduction and dissolution of this conviction, she was able to come out of her feelings of powerlessness and overwhelm and turn to her own life design and desires.

On the basis of a good mentalization of the topic of power and powerlessness, one can decide or look for how one could consciously acquire even more power competence. This can succeed depending on acquired mentalization ability and social competences, e.g. through

- Psychotherapy,
- Discussions,
- Books,
- Family Constellations,
- Seminars,
- Survival Camp,
- Seeking challenges.

Depending on the motivation for power, the spirit of adventure, the will to conquer, the will to master fate, the will to create, the experience of creativity, self-realization, self-love, love of one's neighbor, the measures taken will vary greatly.

▶ Chapter 3 discusses how the concepts of power and powerlessness can be defined and understood, and how the issues of power and powerlessness can be systematically mentalized, in particular which mentalization dimensions should be considered in psychotherapy.

References

Allen JG, Fonagy P, Bateman AW (2011) Mentalisieren in der psychotherapeutischen Praxis. Klett-Cotta, Stuttgart. 2008

Bandura A (1976) Lernen am Modell. Ansätze zu einer sozial-kognitiven Lerntheorie. Klett, Stuttgart

Bandura A (1979) Sozial-kognitive Lerntheorie. Klett-Cotta, Stuttgart
Bischof-Köhler D (2011) Soziale Entwicklung in Kindheit und Jugend—Bindung, empathie, theory of mind. Kohlhammer, Stuttgart
Fonagy P (2003) Bindungstheorie und Psychoanalyse, 3. Aufl. Klett-Cotta, Stuttgart. 2009
Fonagy P, Target M (1998) Ein interpersonelles Verständnis des Säuglings. In: Hurry A (Hrsg) (2002) Psychoanalyse und Entwicklungsförderung von Kindern. Brandes & Apsel, Frankfurt a.M., S. 11–42
Fonagy P, Target M (2006) Psychoanalyse und die Psychopathologie der Entwicklung. Klett-Cotta, Stuttgart
Fonagy P, Gergely G, Jurist E, Target M (2004a) Affektregulierung, Mentalisierung und die Entwicklung des Selbst. Klett-Cotta, Stuttgart
Fonagy P, Gergely G, Jurist EL, Target M (2004b) Entwicklungsaufgaben der normalen Adoleszenz und adoleszenter Zusammenbruch. In: Fonagy P, Gergely G, Jurist EL, Target M (2004) Affektregulierung, Mentalisierung und die Entwicklung des Selbst. Klett-Cotta, Stuttgart, S. 320–342
Freud S (1920) Jenseits des Lustprinzips. GW XIII, S. 1–69
Gergely G, Watson J (1996) Die Theorie des sozialen Biofeedbacks durch mütterliche Affektspiegelung. Selbstpsychologie 17(18):143–194
Gergely G, Watson J (1999) Early social-emotional development: Contingency perception and the social biofeedback model. In: Rachat P (ed) Early social cognition: understanding others in the first months of life. Erlbaum, Hillsdale, NJ, pp 101–137
Gilligan C (1983) Die verlorene Stimme. Campus, Frankfurt a.M.
Goleman D (2008) Soziale Intelligenz. Knaur, München
Hinsch R, Pfingsten U (2007) Das Gruppentraining sozialer Kompetenzen (GSK). Grundlagen, Durchführung, Materialien. Beltz, Weinheim
König K (2008) Brüder und Schwestern. Geburtenfolge als Schicksal, 14. Aufl. Vandenhoeck & Ruprecht, Göttingen
Kohlberg L (1974) Zur kognitiven Entwicklung des Kindes. Suhrkamp, Baden-Baden
Konrad K, Firk C, Uhlhaas PJ (2013) Hirnentwicklung in der Adoleszenz. Dtsch Ärzteblatt 25:425–431
Reddy V (2008) How infants know minds. Harvard University Press, London
Sohni H (2011) Geschwisterdynamik. Psychosozial-Verlag, Gießen
Sowarka B (1995) Soziale Intelligenz und soziale Kompetenz. In: Sarges W (Hrsg) Management-Diagnostik. Hogrefe, Göttingen, S. 365–382
Steinbeis N, Bernhardt BC, Singer T (2012) Impulse control and underlying functions of the left DLPFC mediate age-related and age-independent individual differences in strategic social behavior. Neuron 73(5):1040–1051
Stangl W (2001) Der Begriff der sozialen Kompetenz in der psychologischen Literatur (Version 2.0). p@psych e-zine 3. Jg. http://paedpsych.jk.uni-linz.ac.at/PAEDPSYCH/SOZIALEKOMPETENZ/. (Zuletzt gesehen: 28.02.2016)
Zimbardo PH (2007) Der Luzifer-Effekt. Spektrum-Verlag, Heidelberg, p 2008

Power and Powerlessness: What Is It?

Contents

M.-L. Althoff, *Mentalizing Power and Powerlessness*,
https://doi.org/10.1007/978-3-662-66119-2_3

In this chapter, the basis for a conceptual understanding of power and powerlessness will be established. Based on the Weber's definition of power (extended by Luhmann), various aspects, identifying features and manifestations of power and powerlessness will be discussed. In psychotherapy we are constantly confronted and engaged with power structures of external and internal reality and also experience the challenges of our own involvement in power and powerlessness fantasies and scenarios. In order to be able to come to a reflective and empathic understanding and handling of these challenges ourselves and together with our patients, it will be developed how the topics of power and powerlessness can be mentalized systematically, i.e. which dimensions can be considered and felt, with reference to the theory of mentalization presented in ► Chap. 2.

3.1 Understanding the Concept of Power

Power is an everyday phenomenon in our modern society. Everyone has contact with it, and social and world political order seems inconceivable without power. Yet this has not always been the case. Arno Gruen (2016) suggests that there is evidence of a direct link between the attachment and care of the mother and primary caregivers and the development of empathy, as well as the simultaneous conception of benevolent and benevolent deities in the early days of humanity. Only with the emergence of the "great" cultures about 40,000 years ago and the spread of possessive thinking had the understanding of maternal care and bonding as a phase to be limited and consequently also the limitedness of empathic possibilities as well as the idea of God changed: "the later gods of fear, damnation, and vengeance arguably emerged only with the rise of 'great' civilizations that needed the obedience of their subjects to enforce their claims to rule. Fear and punishment are the means to enforce obedience" (Gruen 2016, p. 57).

Power is as "good" or as "bad" for us as we judge its use, but today we cannot imagine a world without power. The German word "Macht" comes from the Gothic "magan" and originally meant a possibility in the sense of volitional capacity or ability. The English word "power" comes from the latin word potis which means able, capable, possible.

▪ As the Original Enablement

"The state is a community of equal citizens for the purpose of enabling them to lead their best lives." (Aristotle 384-322, Politics)

▪ As the Power of Agency of an Individual

According to Hannah Arendt, this power is conferred and thus legitimized by a group of people who are of one opinion, power being in itself non-violent (Arendt 1963).

▪ As a Temporary Option

"Power does not really belong to anyone; it arises between people when they act together, and it disappears as soon as they disperse again." (Habermas 1981, p. 238f)

As a Revolutionary Possibility

"Those who have understood how power is won and exercised can use this knowledge for purposes of overthrow. The damned of this earth have only to expel the powerful from their magnificent palaces, let the monks preach for them from the pulpits, and everything is already turns topsy-turvy." (Machiavelli 1513, Il Principe)

As a Physical Force

Hobbes sees power in the sense that the state cannot commit injustice because it has the power to make law. (T. Hobbes 1642, De Cive)

As the Realization of Divine Natural Law

According to John Locke, the power of the state serves the realization of human existence and must not be directed against man. (J. Locke 1689, Two Treatises of Government)

As Superiority or Will to Power

"Fear (negative) and the will to power (positive) explain our strong regard for people's opinions" (Nietzsche, Nachlass 1876/77). Nietzsche thinks that in enduring the terrible and cruel of life, the capacity for "tragic greatness" is revealed. First of all, this means an acceptance of fate. Nietzsche, however, demands a further step: one should want fate. Only then does one not merely accept it passively as something imposed, but can integrate it beneficially into the interpretation of one's own life through the act of willing: "Willing liberates: that is the true doctrine of will and freedom" (Nietzsche 1980, p. 111). The "will to power" that is to be concretized in the superman is thus not the will to dominate others, but is to be understood as the will to be able, to enrich oneself, to overcome oneself.

As a Belligerent Confrontation

Michel Foucault describes power relations, but he makes a clear distinction between violence and power: "A relation of violence acts on a body, acts on things: it forces, it bends, it breaks, it destroys: it excludes all possibilities; it is left with no other counterpole than that of passivity. And when it encounters a resistance, it has no choice but to force it down. A power relation, on the other hand, is built on two elements without which no power relation can come into being: so that the 'other' (on whom it acts) remains recognized and preserved as the subject of action until the end, and a whole field of possible responses, reactions, effects, inventions opens up before the power relation. (…) but it is always a way of acting on one or more acting subjects, and this insofar as they act or are capable of acting. An acting upon acts." (Foucault 1987, p. 254f)

As Intersubjective Will Enforcement

Max Weber's classic definition of the term is: "Power means any chance to assert one's own will within a social relationship, even against opposition, regardless of what this chance is based on." (Weber 1922, p. 50)

As a Symbolically Generalized Medium

Power is understood as modal in the sense of a symbolically generalized medium of communication alongside money, love, art, truth, faith, which is influenced by both the powerful and the usurpated (Luhmann 1975). Luhmann's definition of power emphasizes an aspect that goes beyond Weber's definition: according to Luhmann, power is also exercised when someone wanted to act that way anyway and then experiences: He must act this way, his will is irrelevant.

As an Ontological and Social Phenomenon

From a constructivist perspective, it must be stated that man, as an informationally closed system, can only construct information in the course of his self-organization. Then Bateson's approach (1996) is compelling when he concludes that power is merely a very dangerous myth or mythical abstraction and thus "it is (…) epistemological bullshit" which "inevitably leads to various kinds of catastrophes" (Bateson 1996, p. 625). Portele also follows this line of argument when he postulates that "we are involved in the production of power: through power, through obedience, and through our discourses on power and obedience" (Portele and Roessler 1994, p. 143f) and that without the willingness to submit, to servitude, (…) "power cannot be exercised" (Portele 1989, p. 204). He goes on to say that this submission can only be thought of as an autonomous act because of the operational closedness of cognitive systems. "It is on this autonomous decision to give up one's will that the exerciser of power depends. Without this abandonment of his own will, he cannot exercise power." (ibid., p. 206) These statements relegate power to the realm of myths, and it seems that powerlessness is the exclusive responsibility of the powerless. In my view, neither a position that assigns responsibility solely to the powerful, nor a position that views power only as a social construct for which the powerless are responsible, allows for an adequate description of interpersonal phenomena. The first position negates the individual's own responsibility, while the second position negates the responsibility of the powerful. Kraus (2002) suggests that it is necessary to overcome the common "either-or logic" in favour of a "both/and logic". It can neither be claimed that power exists per se nor that it is only constructed; rather, power can be explained both as an ontological and as a social phenomenon.

As Part of the Interaction Process

Böllinger (2008, p. 441) describes power as a socially produced and perceived, action-relevant aspect of the social interaction process. He starts—like many current psychological contributions on power—from Max Weber's definition. According to Böllinger, this definition is neutral because it leaves out any morality to the power holder or the legitimacy of power. Power, according to Böllinger, "expresses itself in manifold and interactively constituted relations of domination as well as in social inter- and intrasystemic as well as interpersonal and intrapsychic conflicts" (ibid., p. 445). Following this idea, the phenomenon of power is thus expressed in particular in psychotherapeutic individual, group and family therapies.

In psychotherapy the phenomenon of power can refer to different areas and dimensions, e.g. to

- yourself: Do I or do I not want what I can? Can I do what I want?
- the choice of words: It sometimes expresses not only the freedom of action of the power holder, but also the ability to do anything at all. Something is "doable" or is "done" one way or another, to the point that there are "feasibility studies". Many training participants begin by asking, "How do I do this, that I achieve the agreed upon goals with the patient?"
- one's own knowledge: The idea that one's knowledge gives power over the course of events, the achievement of goals.
- the technology and the environmental conditions: Can I handle the situation?
- my fellow human being(s): This aspect refers to a relational notion of power, namely the power to cause the other to do what I want (Fink-Eitel 1992). Can I influence others? Can I influence or even dominate others even without words, for example by leaving someone alone or by not leaving?
- to the symbolic-metaphysical realm: the power of fate, the power of feelings, the power of nature, the power of words, the power of myths, etc. is experienced by everyone more or less often. Which forces have power over me?
- Fear of the other: How much power do I grant the other person over me? Hermann Hesse wrote: "If you fear someone, it is because you have granted that someone power over you" (Hesse 1987, p. 40). In this respect, power does not have to be exercised in real terms, it only has to be acknowledged. One must break away from the classical view of power as coercive or violent, for power does not always have to be actively or bilaterally exercised, thus a subordinate to power can also act in the sense of the exerciser of power even before the power is exercised or threatened, in order to circumvent an exercise of power that he has fantasized or anticipated.
- the political environment: How does the power of politics affect me? How strong does the will to power, the striving for power, power behaviour in the sense of acquiring, maintaining and expanding power of each participant appear? Power expansion and power maintenance are central positions in politics and fundamental mechanisms in political action. In social institutions and orders, power serves to ensure that social goals can be realized. In doing so, all elements of the system are supposed to agree to the basic consensus and thus also legitimize the power relations through recognition or acquiescence. Every psychotherapist who offers psychotherapy financed by health health insurances must confirm with every application to a health insurance that he or she complies with the regulations.

3.2 Understanding the Concept of Powerlessness

Powerlessness can also, but not completely, be understood as the opposite of power.

On a physical level, fainting refers to a disturbance of consciousness that is brief and caused by a temporary lack of oxygen to the brain and is usually not life-threatening, but can be damaging due to injuries that occur as a result. **On a psychological level,** powerlessness refers to a state of powerlessness and helplessness that may be experienced permanently in a particular situation or as a result of enduring circumstances. Psychic powerlessness and helplessness can be consciously experienced and processed or unconsciously repressed and (possibly symptomatically) processed. For example, it may be expressed physically as conversion symptomatology (to the point of epileptic-like seizures), or it may be denied to oneself in projective identification onto others. Because of this possible interaction of physical and psychological levels, the physical and psychological levels must always be considered when looking at powerlessness.

Hannah Arendt (1963) sums up this interplay when she writes in Truth and Politics:

> From this perspective, which is essentially oriented towards the conflict between politics and truth, it looks as if politics is about nothing other than struggles for power and interests, as if there were a public space in human coexistence at all only because the necessities of life force people to organize themselves and, as the case may be, to act with or fight each other, in short, as if politics could be defined as the game in which decisions are made.—"Who gets what, when, how?" [Note: Arendt alludes here to the subtitle of a then famous 1936 book by Harold D. Lasswell]. (Arendt 1963, p. 355)

Arendt argues that it is in the nature of things that as soon as one approaches the political realm from the standpoint of truth, especially if one focuses on the problem of factual truth, one does not even get to see what actually constitutes political life—"not the high joy, which is inherent in the sheer coming together with one's peers, not the satisfaction of acting together and the satisfaction of appearing in public, not the possibility, so decisive for all human existence, of intervening in the world by speaking and acting and of creating a new beginning" (ibid., p. 356). Rather, from her point of view of contemplation it emerges,

> that this space, despite its size, is limited, that it does not encompass the totality of human existence, nor the totality of what occurs in the world. What limits it are the things that human beings cannot change, that are beyond their power, and that can only be made to temporarily disappear through lying self-deception. (ibid.)

Following this thought, I would like to include with my reflections on the concept of powerlessness the dimension that concerns the "deprived of one's own power", the "powerless", the "not producible by humans".

In order to be able to look at the human being's feelings of power and powerlessness in this deep dimension from the very beginning, I adopt a developmental psychological perspective, taking into account the psychodynamic and primary therapeutic view and insights into brain development and ontogenetic development (Rank (1924), Grof, Janov, Janus, Chamberlain, Hüter and Weser, among others).

Before I start, however, I would like to make an important remark: The following reflections and insights are not referenced in order to establish how things would be right (and thus all other experiences would be wrong and inferior), but rather the aim is to think and feel our way into soul life at the time of first experiences of powerlessness, in order to understand what *can* possibly lead to certain difficulties or experiences later in life, and how we can intervene and change, or what we must accept and embrace. My belief is:

> No one can grow up in an ideal state, not everything can be controlled (illnesses, death, accidents, alcohol consumption before knowing pregnancy). Mothers and fathers can only be who they can be. And even if everything were feasible, it could also not be expected that everything would then be peaceful and harmonious.

Possibly, however, we can expect to recover something of the care and nurturance of earlier "primitive" cultures more than 40,000 years past by incorporating the fact that the baby is a sentient being from the beginning, even before birth, and by the empathy this makes possible for us (cf. Gruen 2016).

3.2.1 Hypotheses on the Experience of Powerlessness of a Baby

The experience of powerlessness can be divided into three phases according to the development of the brain.

The First Level of Consciousness (Cerebellum)

The first level of consciousness is localized in the cerebellum or brain stem. This part of the brain is a very old part of the brain that is also present in reptiles and is therefore also called the reptilian brain. The development of this first level of the brain begins at conception and ends a few weeks after birth. Although the midbrain and the bar also form by the 15th fetal week of life, and the cerebral hemispheres also begin to grow rapidly, the neurons are not yet fully formed and are poorly interconnected. Thus, the brain is still quite immature at the time of birth. Only the brain stem is already completely interconnected. This circumstance explains that an infant shortly after birth does not yet have tears (although it can feel). It can be understood in this way that "the infant is"—it is what it's system receives from the outside world, and cannot yet oppose it. When there is a tension of need, the infant is the pain caused by the deficits in his system. The infant at this time is entirely the state of his being; it cannot distance itself from itself and from what is happening to him (in relation to its life-needs). It cannot interpret it as good or bad or temporary; it *is* simply that state.

▪ The Needs and the Experience of Powerlessness of the First Level

So the embryo or the baby *is*, and there are **needs from the beginning**, for example, to have enough oxygen. Having oxygen available is normally ensured by the mother being healthy, not smoking, not drinking alcohol, eating a healthy diet and having little emotional stress.

The baby initiates birth because—according to researchers—it has the **need to be born**. The baby secretes certain hormones that are absorbed by the placenta.

Now it has the need **for labor to begin**, not too weak and not too strong, just right and in tune with its strength. During birth it has the **need for sufficient oxygen**. (To go into the individual phases of birth or perinatal matrices (Grof 1975) would go too far here).

The **needs after birth are** well known: Safety, protection, warmth, physical contact, the mother's breast, her heartbeat, her voice. So what was always there and familiar in the belly can be found again. And yet the infant often feels the **need to cry**.

In relation to the experience of powerlessness, we can assume that the non-fulfillment of needs at a certain point means pain. Not being able to react to the pain itself in such a way that the state changes means powerlessness.

These experiences that an embryo or baby has from conception until a few weeks after birth become hard-coded experiences in the brain stem that provide an experiential base for everything to come. It is often asked why pain is stored in the body. Wouldn't it be better if these experiences, similar to action sequences, were not stored due to immature storage capabilities? In the same way, one can ask why fear at birth should become an initial fear.

So what is the point of the body storing pain? Perhaps it is that these experiences are stored because they want to heal again. Or maybe they activate physical pain later in life when the person does not recognize their psychological problems (Upledger 1996). But perhaps this circumstance is simply due to the fact that the baby initially has no way of distinguishing which experiences should be stored and which should not. When it comes to adaptation to the environment, the organism learns to survive. Janov mentions an elementary principle according to which "every intrusion or foreign force in living organisms produces a biological structure that can cope with it" (Janov 1981, p. 319).

A picture (Janov 1993) helps to understand this evolutionary principle: An amoeba lives in water. The amoeba lives willy-nilly in this water, because otherwise it must die. Imagine putting an amoeba as an experimental animal in water that has been contaminated with ink. The amoeba accepts the contamination for lack of an alternative. The experiment leaders now register that the amoeba has the ability to filter the ink particles out of the water and store them in its cell body until it has the opportunity to get rid of the ink in the water.

In a figurative sense, the embryo or baby has needs and depends on these needs being met in order to survive, just as the amoeba needs water. Desires that are not fulfilled and cause pain correspond to the unusable, superfluous ink that is stored. First of all, however, the water does not exist without ink; in the same way, the infant does not have the choice to absorb only good experiences and store them as a foundation.

As already mentioned, it is impossible to meet all the needs of the embryo or the baby. Pregnancy and birth are subject to a variety of internal and external conditions which, in a figurative sense, can "muddy the waters" in many ways, e.g. accidents, illnesses, marital crises, natural disasters, terror, war etc.

The embryo, the baby cannot protect itself, is enclosed in its world, cannot react effectively (or its reactions are not even noticed), is at the mercy. This state can be interpreted as a powerless experience. Situations of early powerlessness are given when e.g.

- the mother's body at birth does not respond to the fetal signals,
- the umbilical cord is around the neck or over the shoulder and no one notices,
- the pelvis is too narrow and all the baby's efforts to get out are useless.

It is well known that birth can become a traumatic experience for the infant (and the mother) for many reasons. This cannot always be prevented either, but the **baby's need to cry** becomes **all** the more existential. At its best, after all its vital needs for food, warmth, and rest are met, the baby can cry out the pain of its history, in the arms of its mother, father, or caregiver. And there is nothing wrong with it and does not question the parents, they have not, as they often fear, "failed"—on the contrary.

To speak in analogy to the amoeba image, the loving arms in which the baby is held when it cries out its pain are the "water", and the pain it has experienced is the cached "ink" that can now be excreted by its crying. But if the crying baby is left alone—without the attention of a caregiver—new pain is likely to develop, the feeling of abandonment and loneliness. More and more "ink" has to be absorbed and cached, so to speak. As a result, the feeling of being "alone in the world" arises, feelings of loneliness, abandonment and self-alienation and powerlessness arise, and the feeling that nothing can be done about it. It may have just been scared to death and was already blue because it was stuck in the pelvis and couldn't breathe. Now it's lying in a small bed without the familiar and comforting sounds of its mother's heartbeat and voice, and it's loud and glaring and strange. And then when it falls asleep exhausted, you just can't say, "Oh, how peacefully it sleeps!"

Powerlessness is born, in every case. But the extent to which we experience powerlessness determines how exposed we experience ourselves later in life and how much we have to suppress, project or deny an experience of pain and powerlessness. When our needs are ignored and there is nothing we can do to meet them—how do we cope? You know that feeling of being faced with a situation and not being able to do anything? What do you **do** then? Do you endure it? Well, as a baby you endured it; you had no choice. Probably the more you felt held as a child, the better you hold out **powerlessness (= not being able to do anything = not having any power)**, unless there were other traumatic events.

Panksepp (2003), for example, has generally demonstrated that pain and suffering are relieved by the support and loving attention of others. He also suggests that, conversely, denial and suppression of pain prevents the release of opioids, especially endorphins, and therefore, if pain is not relieved, the conditions for violent aggression and the permanent suppression of compassion are created. Gruen even goes so far as to see this as a central reason for the emergence of warlike cultures:

> » The neurochemistry of social bonding shows that the despair over separateness that accompanies disruption of mother-infant bonding produces the pain of loss of social support, and this distinguishes peaceful cultures from warring cultures of conquest. (Gruen 2016, p. 79)

These connections are so worth considering that I would like to elaborate a little further here: the human body is known to be able to produce endogenous drugs under certain circumstances. These endogenous opioids (more precisely: opioid peptides) are also called endorphins. Without endorphins, the mother's immune system would reject the embryo as a foreign body, i.e. foreign protein. For this reason, the bloodstream of the mother and the baby contains an increased concentration of endorphins during pregnancy and until birth. Our first "addictive substance", the endorphins, therefore make life possible in the first place. At the latest after birth, the baby is cut off from this source. If the infant is breastfed by the mother, it continues to receive a morphine-like substance through the mother's milk, which makes it possible for it to go into "withdrawal" a little more gently. It is reasonable to assume that a breastfed baby can cope with "withdrawal" somewhat better than a bottle-fed baby. But I would like to emphasize that this only covers the physical-biological level for the time being, not the emotional-supply level.

Were there complications during pregnancy, was the mother stressed or depressed, was the birth traumatic, e.g. because the child did not manage to come out under its own power, or because the baby was too big, or because the supply of oxygen was not enough, or because it was already born blue, or even because it had to be resuscitated? All experiences are—as mentioned at the beginning—registered in the brain stem and thus shape behaviour patterns for future life. It is aggravating if life continues to hold hardships in store; it is relieving if the child can already cry out the pain of its traumatic experiences as a baby in safety and security.

There is a connection with the autonomic nervous system. We have two complementary nervous systems: the sympathetic and the parasympathetic nervous system. The sympathetic nervous system ensures that the body reacts optimally under stress. By releasing certain hormones such as adrenaline, the sympathetic nervous system serves to increase performance in emergency situations. The counterpart of the sympathetic nervous system is the parasympathetic nervous system. It serves the metabolism and the build-up of physical reserves in the resting state of the body. Janov (1993, 2000) postulates that people can be classified into one of these categories, the group of "sympathetics" and that of "parasympathetics". According to him, if a baby is born and the "parasympathetic" nervous system has been in action, it will develop into a "parasympathetic" and vice versa.

Schore (1994) also discusses these different personality types. He informs that this distinction was already described in 1915:

> » The study of personality differences in the psychophysiological expression of emotional behavior can be traced back to the work of Eppinger and Hess (1915), who discovered that individuals fell into two distinct category types with respect to their psychopharmacological response to sympathetic and parasympathetic active substances, respectively, differing in their physiological response to autonomic system stress. A "sympatheticotonic" type was characterized by dominance of sympathetic responses such as rapid heartbeat, enlarged pupils, and easily aroused temperament. A second "vagotonic" pattern reflected an increased disposition (a tendency) to react with the vagus nerve and the parasympathetic branch of the autonomic nervous system, reflected in low heart rate and small pupils. (Schore 1994, p. 278)

But whereas, according to Janov's theory, the birth experience essentially determines the personality type (which is then either mitigated or reinforced later in life), Schore (referring to many other authors) justifies the emergence of different physiological and psychological character traits exclusively by different early experiences of the infant with the attachment figures during the first two years of life. He does not describe birth and prenatal influences at all. In my view, both aspects should be considered or taken into account in therapeutic work. For our consideration of early powerlessness I still remain with the consideration of the early experience of the baby.

Imagine a baby sliding down the birth canal and its umbilical cord tightening around the neck. The further it slides down the birth canal, the tighter the cord tightens; the oxygen becomes less. Now the brain receives the message that further exertion is life-threatening, the previously active sympathetic nervous system is deactivated and the parasympathetic nervous system takes over. If this state continues for a long time, the baby's oxygen is reduced from the outside to the inside, which means: first the limbs, then the vital organs come under oxygen deficiency, and then only the brain is supplied with oxygen.

Example in which birth experience plays a role: A patient had the thought of hanging himself. In a therapy session he felt how he could no longer breathe, how everything was constricting and he could do nothing at all about it. Taking one's own life means going into the **power to** kill oneself in order to finally be able to do something (cf. Janov 2007).

If everything goes normally, the birth is triggered by the baby or its hormonal impulse, it "knows" the date. If the baby is then born, while the sympathetic nervous system was active, it has the feeling of having "made it". It becomes easier to develop a feeling and a conviction that effort is worthwhile and that one can trust one's impulses. However, if it has been very strenuous, an exaggerated "life is struggle from the beginning" may also form as an unconscious belief and emotional readiness.

If the baby sees the light of day while the parasympathetic nervous system was active, it probably has a feeling of "not having made it" or "being rescued or fetched at the last moment", e.g. with a suction cup, caesarean section or pressing on the mother's belly from the outside. It has experienced that it could **do** nothing, that effort is of no use or life-threatening. It may internalize that one should not trust its impulses. Everything that interferes with the birth process is registered by the brain as pain or terror, not being able to do anything as powerlessness. Powerlessness and terror are equal in strength, because at this stage we cannot yet speak of feelings in the proper sense, because feelings run through the limbic system, the midbrain, which is not yet sufficiently differentiated. In view of these considerations, it is thought-provoking that more and more children—for various reasons—are "delivered" by caesarean section. In the USA, doctors often have to pay high damages after charges and civil suits, which is an expression of parental "powerlessness", to which the doctors then react with a planned birth and thus the threatening "powerlessness" seems to be overcome.

After birth, the baby—in the negative case—lies alone in his crib and cries:

- If it is hungry, it cannot go to the fridge, but has to wait screaming until the given (breast-)feeding time is reached.
- When its cold, it can't put on a warm blanket or find someone to snuggle with, but has to wait, screaming, for someone to come up with the idea that (human) warmth might be missing.
- When it is thirsty, it cannot open a bottle, but has to wait screaming until diaper changing, blanket changing has been tried.
- When there are too many noises and lights, it has to wait, screaming, for someone to pick it up and comfort it.

It is completely at the mercy of everything. The baby cries because it needs to get rid of its frustration. Crying alone—as already mentioned—is by no means good according to the motto "Crying is healthy and strengthens the lungs!". This completely misjudges the baby's neediness and loads it with new pain. It is not understood, and it cannot do anything about it: experience of powerlessness upon experience of powerlessness.

▶ Example

One patient who had problems with drinking came to the realization that he wanted to numb his powerlessness with alcohol and that there was a direct connection with a feeling of being constricted and his drinking. That was all he could **do** as a baby, drink! ◀

The Second Level of Consciousness (Midbrain)

The second level of consciousness is called the midbrain or the middle level of the limbic system. Strictly speaking, the limbic system is not a spatially delimited area of the brain, but a functional unit.

▪ Lower Level

The lower level of the limbic system regulates the bodily functions and behaviors that are essential for survival, and it communicates with the cerebellum. Thus, the triggering and control of innate behaviors such as flight, freezing, attack, stress regulation, and elementary affective-emotional states such as fear/fright, anger/rage, joy/comfort, disgust, interest, or sadness occur here. It is also responsible for the release of endorphins.

▪ Middle Level

At the middle level, the level of our momentary observation, unconscious processes of emotion emergence, differentiation and control, behavioral evaluation and conditioning are located (Roth and Strüber 2014).

▪ Upper Level

The upper level, the limbic level formed by areas of the cerebral cortex, is related to conscious feelings and motives, but also to socialization.

The development and regulation of emotion and drive behaviour must therefore always be seen as the interaction of many parts of the brain, whereby the limbic system must be attributed a central evaluation function. Modern neuroscience therefore refers to the limbic system as an emotional power centre in the brain (Häusel 2008). Roth and Strüber (2014) refer to the limbic system in its function as a switch board as the "seat of the psychic".

The development of emotional differentiation begins after birth (and is completed with integration of the different modes by the 5th/6th year of life; cf. stages of mentalization development). When the baby sheds tears, this is a sign that it feels pain as pain and differentiates it from other states. From now on it can feel and consequently suffer. So the baby **is** no longer the pain or suffering as at the first level, but now it **feels** the pain, it suffers. But it does not yet **know** consciously that it is suffering, the cerebrum is not yet developed enough for that.

▪ The Needs and the Experience of Powerlessness of the Second Level

At this level, too, the child naturally has needs beyond those of the first level (such as food, clothing, security, safety, warmth, attention, stimulation and attention). There is also the need for at least one permanent caregiver. Without at least one reliable caregiver, the infant has difficulty developing emotionally. This also means that the limbic system may develop in an unfavorable manner. The child's need for emotional **attachment** and reference is so great that the child accepts everything, i.e. care, safety, love, protection, security in the good case and disregard, beatings, mistreatment, sexual abuse in the bad case.

The baby and toddler also has no choice at first—just like the foetus and infant. It takes what it gets, because its needs are vital and it has no means of comparison. What it experiences is "normal" for the child; it does not "deserve" anything else in its own imagination, because no alternatives are conceivable or contained in its horizon of experience. It relates everything to itself.

The child initially understands only emotionally; the neocortex is not yet mature enough. It is known that for this reason a child cannot consciously lie until the age of 5. If it tells the untruth—in the eyes of adults—this happens out of an emotional feeling, e.g. fear. For example, it sees the threatening, angry look on it's mother's or father's face and reacts fearfully in the negative to questions. If the child's fear of its caregiver is even justified, the result is a relationship disturbed by anxiety stress that in no way meets the child's needs. These conditions usually have an unfavorable effect on the further development of the limbic system.

Extreme examples have become known in which offenders show no remorse, in which the impression is created that "cold-blooded" action was taken. Empathy for the victim is not possible for the offender, he seems "untouched". This behavior is a sure sign that the limbic system and consequently the mentalization ability could only develop insufficiently.

Of course, it is impossible to meet all the needs of the child at all times. Parents are not perfect and have needs too. Some frustration at this stage of development can also contribute to a healthy subject-object differentiation. And children also begin to develop their own theories and defense strategies at this age, which they then use to (unconsciously) feel powerful. The less security is experienced, the more the split-off feelings of powerlessness can turn into feelings of power. In this respect, it is important that the caregivers allow the child to express his or her emotions, e.g. by crying or temper tantrums about the frustration of his or her needs. Should the child not be able to let out his pain in the experience of security, it is possible that the child's experience confirms what it learned as a baby on the first level. The child is shaped by the first level experiences. If the crying is suppressed, if its outbursts are punished, if it receives beatings for its fits of raving madness, then not only can its system not heal, but it experiences even more pain in addition to the suffering that already exists.

Examples like the following are many: In response to a child's crying, parents try to figure out why he or she is crying. If they can't find an understandable reason, they may say, "Stop it already. You have no reason to cry."

- Increase 1: "You're already a big girl/boy. Stop it!"
- Increase 2: "Go to your room and don't come back until you calm down."
- Increase 3: "Crying won't help you either, it will only make it worse."
- Increase 4: "If you don't stop right now, we'll give you reason to cry."
- Increase 5: "Do you want me to smack you so you know why you're crying?"

The powerlessness that the parents experience in the face of the crying child is turned into power—the child will also learn, internalize and use this—and sometimes this power is discharged in the form of violence. It is likely that in such situations the parents act and react out of helplessness, but also out of the activation of their own pain body. In this respect, it is so incredibly important that adults are aware of their own pain body and have a sense of when it is activated. In the best case scenario, the healing of one's pain body should have already begun. (These considerations also apply to psychotherapists in dealing with their patients).

The child, however, whose body was in the process of healing with the crying, because it began to let out the pain, feels misunderstood and abandoned. It cannot do anything with its feelings now, possibly feels wrong or inappropriate, it does not understand itself or cannot explain anything because its mind is not yet developed accordingly. Powerlessness rises, possibly accompanied by great anger. It feels emotionally abandoned and also alienated from itself.

Depending on the experience at its first level, the child will now behave: The "sympathetic" will not stop crying and will defy, lash out, express anger at the parents. The "parasympathetic" resigns because he has learned that reacting and working against can be dangerous and possibly even fatal. This is where the formation of a false self can occur (e.g., Winnicott 1965; Miller 1979; Gruen 1984; Fonagy et al. 2004).

In either case, the child feels confused, abandoned, and powerless. Gruen (1984) sees it as a task of therapy to uncover and liberate a person's original autonomy. He criticizes classical psychoanalysis in this context:

> This is what Oedipus really embodies: the original hurt that turns into the pursuit of dominance (…). What is often considered to be working through an Oedipus complex (…) is the liberation from scruples, the reinforcement of ambition, competition and power. (Gruen 1984, p. 17f)

In my opinion, the liberation from scruples, the reinforcement of ambition, competition and power cannot only be held against psychoanalysis. In psychotherapies of all methods, one sometimes has the impression that from a wrongly or superficially understood promotion of autonomy, egocentrics emerge who are still alienated from themselves.

> The deep hurts that lead to feelings of unacceptable helplessness and anxiety cannot really be touched in a therapy that is wedded to the ideology of domination and power. (ibid.)

The Third Level of Consciousness (Cerebrum)

The development of the third level (the cerebrum or neocortex) proceeds rapidly from the age of 3 years. The overproduction and selection of synapses occur in different regions of the brain at different speeds and intensities and at different times. In the occipital lobe (visual perception), the highest density of synapses is reached in the first months of life. In contrast, growth in the frontal lobe (thinking and planning, judgment, attention) is greatest between the 3rd and 6th year of life. From around the 5th/6th year of life, a child is able to lie consciously and in a planned manner.

After age 6, brain development generally slows until it is complete by age 18, although plasticity is known to remain.

In the networking of the neocortex, the upper limbic level formed by areas of the cerebral cortex plays a major role, as already mentioned. According to Roth and Strüber (2014), this level enables impulse inhibition and reward deferral, frustration tolerance, empathy, reflection, goal setting, and planning for future action. This upper level is about cognitively explaining the world and finding justifications for one's behavior. This is also where conscious emotional-social learning takes place. In addition, the emotional reactions of the two lower limbic levels are strengthened or weakened here, depending on how the demands of socialisation were or are. Evaluations at this level form the basis for the development of morality, ethics, ideas about family, friendship, love, and attitudes toward profit and success-seeking. These developments occur in late childhood and adolescence on the basis of social-emotional experiences.

▪ The Needs and the Experience of Powerlessness of the Third Level

The needs at this level continue to be safety, protection, warmth, physical contact, attention, love, at least one permanent caregiver, as well as trust, freedom, space, other caregivers, friends, education. The more self-confident a child has been able to develop, the more actively he or she will already be able to strive to fulfil needs or to work for them.

The acquired defense mechanisms help the child to be able to find its place in the family, school and circle of friends. The defense mechanisms enable the child to escape the pain of the first and second level. I would like to emphasize here explicitly that defense mechanisms are necessary survival mechanisms. Only when a defense formation expresses itself in a disorder or suffering worthy of illness should it be questioned. It becomes possible for the child and adolescent to develop unaware? of pain, since the functioning defence mechanism suppresses the conscious experience of pain at earlier levels.

In the positive case, the child will, for example, try to succeed in school if it realizes that this is important to its parents. Likewise, it will engage in sports if this finds the favor of father or mother. Children try to be and **do** what they are in all likelihood loved for by their parents. In addition, the child can also use its play and free space to relate to other people who are more likely to meet its (current) needs. If this is successful, healthy and solid defence mechanisms (such as intellectualisation, humourisation, sublimation) are formed, which also help the child to find its place in life in the longer term.

In the negative case, however, the child cannot be an unburdened child. As a result, it cannot develop a healthy defensive formation. The possible constellations are numerous, e.g. when

- the child, despite his efforts, does not succeed in being accepted;
- parents, for example, are unpredictable, their moods directly on the child;
- father or mother are alcoholics and quarrels and violence are prevalent in the family;
- the child is even sexually abused by one of the parents;
- constant quarrels between parents leads to divorce;
- one parent is chronically ill and when the other has to go to work;
- both parents are completely absent as caregivers for the child, e.g. due to an accident;
- the child is needed as a partner, as the father or mother of its parents.

What happens is that the body grows, but the development stops in essential aspects, so that the child cannot really grow up and become independent. Depending on the history at the first levels, the feeling of powerlessness is omnipresent. If the child has not been able to develop effective defense mechanisms against the primal pain of previous levels, it will continue to be unable to build up a defense formation despite massive primal pain if the family or social environment continues to be chaotic and/or abusive. Thus it comes to the fact that its defense constructions continue not to function well. Depending on the intensity and nature of the pain, it will be closer to psychosis than neurosis.

This does not mean that the child cannot be intelligent. On the contrary, it may even be highly intelligent (Miller 1979). However, this intelligence thus formed is always also an escape from pain (Miller 2007). Thus, a balance between pain and power can emerge. Depending on the primal pain, the child will take one direction or the other, "super smart" or, on the contrary, "super stupid", up to the point of lack of motivation with regard to learning.

Upon entering puberty, the interconnection of the three brain levels is largely complete. Depending on the developmental possibilities of the three levels, adolescents then have a defense formation that functions well or poorly—in terms of coping with life. For the sake of clarity, I am comparing well and poorly functioning formations; all conceivable combinations of well and less well functioning defence areas also exist, of course.

With a good constellation of defenses, adolescents will confront their parents' values; some will oppose fiercely and challenge parents, but ultimately set themselves on a good path, i.e., finish school, enter vocational training, or go to college. They have contacts and bonds with peers and make plans for their future.

With a poor defensive formation now comes the first self-harm, drug and alcohol abuse and suicidal thoughts or attempts, because now the young people become aware that they are suffering, but they experience themselves as powerless and think there is nothing they can **do** to change this.

- **Example**

One adolescent patient said, "At 12, I didn't know how to end this futility. I tried as hard as possible not to think about it or think about how I could kill myself."

Power and Powerlessness as an Adult

- **The Needs and the Experience of Powerlessness of Adults**

The needs of adults are manifold, but really vital seem to be food, drink, clothing, sleep, safety, contact and possibly sexuality (about this the minds argue, but that is not the point here). Adults often live in the illusion and hope that they can now finally satisfy all their needs or, if necessary, provide for them themselves.

For the following example, I will return to Janov's amoeba picture (1993): Imagine that two people fall in love. The infatuation is also noticeable in the body, because certain messenger substances and hormones are increasingly released, e.g. dopamine, adrenaline and oxytocin. A frenzy-like state of joyful anticipation and high hopes is known to occur. The loved one seems to be all that one needs and has always longed for. One does not see what he or she is "really" like. There is marriage. He or she is in absolute expectation that everything will be fine now, to get "it" now.

We remember the amoeba with the ink! Being loved by a human being is like "finally returning to my natural water". It is postulated that there is a lifelong willingness of the body to want to heal (e.g., findings in nursing homes support this). So the body senses a healing possibility and wants most of all to cry out all pain, i.e. to get rid of the "ink".

In the psychic, however, this need remains unconscious. It is not anchored in our consciousness that at the beginning of a love relationship there may be the need to cry out one's pain in the arms of the beloved person, just as one would have wanted to cry it out in the arms of one's mother or father. Instead of letting this need come to consciousness, one now wants to receive from the partner all that one did not receive on the three levels as baby, toddler, child. This overlooks the fact that you yourself have grown up in the meantime and that your partner cannot fulfil these wishes because he or she has no power to change the past. Perhaps together in the beginning one drinks a lot of alcohol, has a lot of sex and lives a relatively numbed life in which work is just about managed but friends often feel neglected. In this respect, you become as unaware of the powerlessness that has already brewed on both sides as you are of your true needs.

If the infatuation subsides, and this is the case at the latest when the system stops flooding the body with adrenaline (otherwise it would be too exhausting for the system at some point), the "rose-coloured glasses" dissolve. We see the other person as he or she is. In order not to have to feel the disappointment and powerlessness, one looks for a way out, which makes it possible to keep one's own inner pain unconscious. This way out is then to make the partner the culprit. If one does not reflect or discuss with others at this point, one does not come to one's senses. One remains in the conviction, or rather one gets stuck in the conviction, that one's partner owes one everything one longs for: love, security, care, warmth, safety, recognition, material goods. If this cannot be realized, one can break off the relationship out of disappointment (which is often not the worst thing to do if one is the exploited partner), start an affair, build a house, throw oneself into one's job, leave the country, start all over again somewhere else. One can also raise one's supposedly legitimate demands on one's partner higher and higher, or present them more and more violently, or, on the other hand, spend oneself in trying to satisfy these (in all likelihood never-ending) demands, or one can also have children, to which one can attach the hope that everything will now be better (the beginning of a new loop).

But what happens when you can't do all that, when you can't avoid the early pain from the lower levels of the brain that comes up?

▪ Therapy

The affected person must find a suitable therapy in which this pain can be consciously experienced or at least must be acknowledged as existing, otherwise the adult will still not have consciously understood what is happening to him or her (► Chap. 7). To do this, he or she must learn to trust both himself or herself and the therapist. Often it already fails to trust oneself.

▪ Blame

Otherwise there would still be the possibility to blame the partner or to accept that the pain attacks one's own system, which manifests itself in illness. But everything one **does** then seems to be insufficient, because the (early) needs remain unsatisfied. Powerlessness forces its way into consciousness, namely the long forgotten powerlessness.

▪ Unilateral Power

Or the adult goes into the position of power, even before the pain has the slightest chance to be consciously perceived. He or she consciously thinks that he or she is now an adult, that he or she no longer has to put up with everything like a little child, that he or she can defend himself or herself. The size of the power position the adult goes into probably corresponds to the size of the unconscious powerlessness he or she experienced at early levels. Power and inner pain must correspond in size, because otherwise the old pain could penetrate, and it must not, because the repression of the pain was vital in early childhood, but now prevents it from becoming conscious.

▪ Mutual Power

Both partners can also go into the position of power, which can ultimately lead to murder and manslaughter. This is rather the exception, as we know. Usually one partner goes into power and thereby forces the other to go into powerlessness. Then their relationship has probably reached the point where they hate each other, because neither wants to be the way he or she is now, or is seen to be, nor does he or she want to be in the situation he or she is in now.

Power-Powerlessness-Circle

Possibly those affected reinforce their conviction once again and emphasize that the other person must give or change. The supposedly "smarter" one gives in and allows himself or herself to be persuaded to go shopping, go on holiday, do unskilled work, etc. that he or she did not actually want. The more powerful partner forces himself or herself to do what he or she wants, without ever becoming permanently more satisfied as a result. In addition, and this makes a joint solution more difficult, the more powerful partner, if his/her unconscious powerlessness potential is great, may not even be aware of any guilt. He/she usually says in such cases that the partner would have wanted it that way. Often little can be said against this, because in all probability one chooses as a partner the one whose powerlessness has remained powerlessness, others would have left long ago, i.e. it is about someone who even as an adult cannot go into power or whose powerlessness forces him/her into illness. Paradoxically, the illness is then power, thus closing the power-powerlessness circle of the couple—in the sense of a collusion (Willi 1975).

Then there are the adults who can't fall in love and commit in the first place. In our time, it has become more and more acceptable to live a permanently single life, placing one's hopes in a successful professional career. He/she becomes a manager, doctor, politician, professor, psychotherapist, teacher, entrepreneur. And it does not matter then whether it is the money in the profession or the image of the profession that should bring it. The value of the profession promises the power and recognition that unconsciously hold the pain and powerlessness. Again, the greater the unconscious powerlessness, the greater the power that must be built up—even if it ends up being dictatorship or, paradoxically, downfall. Our modern world is characterized by this powerlessness, although we are consciously more and more convinced that we can control everything and have it under control. Jürgen Habermas (1985) points out the destructive power inherent in this unconscious approach:

> Today, the imperatives of business and administration, mediated through the media of money and power, intrude into areas that somehow break down when they are disconnected from communication-oriented action and switched to such media-driven interactions. (Habermas 1985, p. 189)

We have the power as adults to escape the conscious experience of powerlessness. In our society, we almost all do, which is to suppress powerlessness as soon as we sense it. But this suppression of powerlessness and pain comes at a cost. We begin to consume things and relationships we don't need, like addicts in search of feelings of happiness and as a substitute for naturally released endorphins:

- Frustration Shopping,
- eat too much,
- smoke too much,
- too much alcohol,
- addictive sex,
- Work addiction,
- Cleanliness mania.

All the while knowing full well that this is damaging our physical and mental health. The diseases of civilization are well known, and yet we **do** this collectively to suppress the old feelings of our own pain (and those that have accumulated over generations) that want to come up.

> The entire repertoire of acting out our old defenses in the form of addiction-like compulsive acts is under the unconscious collective motto/oath: "Never again be powerless like before!"

In order to understand, experience and change this unconscious oath in psychotherapy, mental work of the individual and in cooperation in psychotherapy is necessary. A recognized effective possibility is that of (jointly) mentalizing an issue to be dealt with. This in itself does not solve any problems, but it first creates the possibility of doing so, because a basis of thoughts and feelings is worked out which can enable the individual or the patient-therapist pair to have established a solid reflected basis for change and decision-making. Last but not least, in a positive case, the view of the world becomes richer and clearer.

3.3 Dimensions of the Mentalization of Power: The Star in Balance

The concept of mentalization encompasses various dimensions of social cognitions. These mentalization dimensions are of course also and even especially valid for the topic of power/powerlessness. Luyten et al. (2011) have formulated four dimensions that allow a clearer, more systematic capture of mentalizing ability in clinical and empirical contexts:

- cognitive vs. affective,
- internal vs. external focus,
- self-oriented vs. other-oriented,
- automatic vs. controlled.

3.3.1 Dimension Cognitive-affective

A differentiation is considered between more cognitive and more affective parts of mentalization. Cognitive aspects are described by the Theory of Mind. The theory of (unconscious) pathogenic beliefs can also be included (Weiss 1993). Affective mentalization (Jurist 2008) concerns the area of identifying, understanding, and regulating affects. The general question of when and to what extent a persistent imbalance of the two parts is more likely to represent a defensive formation or a structural weakness is not settled. Likewise, the ability to mentalize always depends on the specific context and the respective relationship quality. Case vignettes are examined in this book (▶ Chaps. 5 and 6).

3.3.2 Dimension Internal-External

Mentalizing activity can further refer to content that is internal or external in origin. Luyten et al. (2011) distinguish processes that focus on externally readable aspects of the self or others from those that refer to inferences regarding internal mental states. It is noted that the processing of these different sources of information each appear to correspond to different neural correlates. Sapute and Lieberman (2006) postulate that medial prefrontal areas associated with biographical memory process aspects of social cognition that relate to Internal states, whereas frontoparietal brain areas process stimuli that are more likely to target external indicators.

3.3.3 Dimension Self-other

Luyten et al. (2011) distinguish in the third dimension between the focus on oneself and the reference to others. These two foci are not fundamentally different, but rather condition each other. In child development, a self-concept is formed through the reference of others to the child's mental states (ontogenetic aspect). Findings from studies with imaging techniques indicate that the neuronal networks activated during mentalizing about self and others show wide overlapping areas (anatomical aspect). In this respect, it can be assumed that an imbalance in the mentalization of the two poles can be regarded as an etiopathogenetic aspect.

3.3.4 Dimension Automatic (Implicit)-controlled (Explicit)

According to Luyten et al. (2011), implicit-automatic, spontaneous, more reflexive social cognition processes are associated with phylogenetically older neural networks. This refers to the amygdalae, basal ganglia, ventromedial prefrontal cortices, and rostral anterior cingulate cortex.

The explicit-controlled mentalizing activities are assigned to the phylogenetically younger regions of the medial temporal lobes and the medial and lateral prefrontal cortices. These processes are slower because their activation involves processes of meaning-making, goal-directed attention, and conscious registration of mental activity. Explicit mentalization processes can be stimulated by the psychotherapist in psychotherapy.

In a concrete clinical situation, when emotional stress and especially attachment stress are high for the patient, a simple idea of a mentalization star can help the psychotherapist to keep the mentalization dimensions in view (◘ Fig. 3.1 and ► Sect. 5.3).

The therapeutic encounter takes place in a constant interplay—from ascending spontaneous and implicit communication through free association and equal attention to exploration (◘ Fig. 3.2).

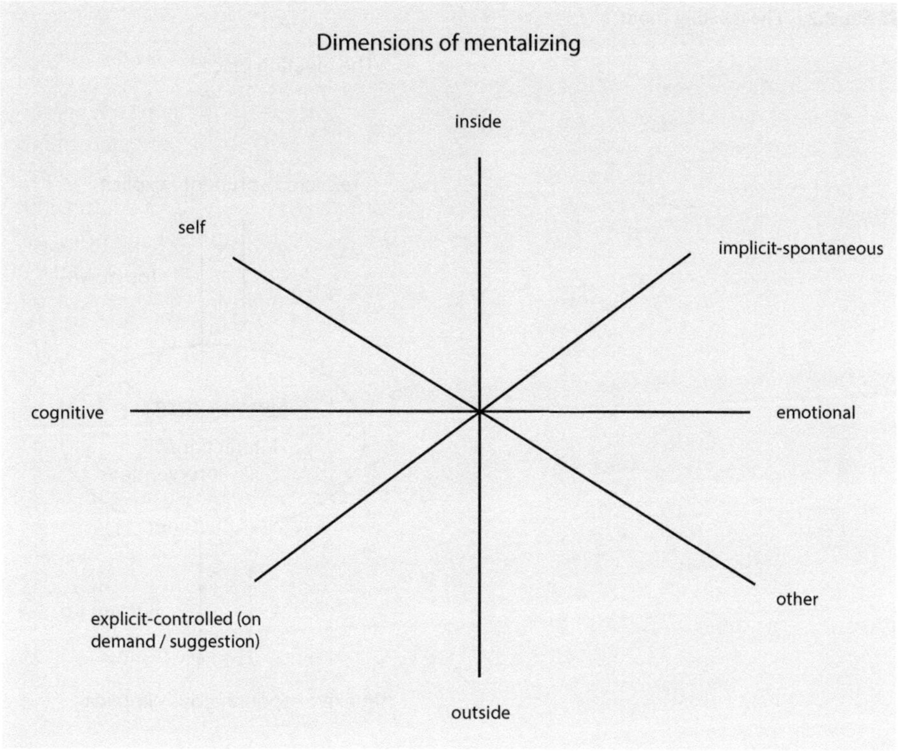

Fig. 3.1 The mentalization star

A normal mentalizing ability is characterized by the fact that there is a balance between the poles of the mentioned mentalizing dimensions. In the case of an unbalanced or polarized mentalizing activity, the mentalizing ability as a whole is assessed as deviant.

3.3.5 Specific Disorders of the Mentalizing Ability

Hypomentalizing (Undermentalizing, Mind-blindness)

This form of deficit mentalizing refers to the situationally unavailable or generally lacking ability to perceive motives and affects of others as well as one's own motives and affects. The general lack of ability is found, for example, in Asperger's syndrome (cf. Schultz-Venrath 2013).

Hypermentalizing (Pseudomentalizing, Overmentalizing, Pretend-mode)

In the state of hypermentalism, motives and affects are ascribed to others or these are exaggerated excessively. Motives and affects are also interpreted into oneself

Fig. 3.2 The meeting room

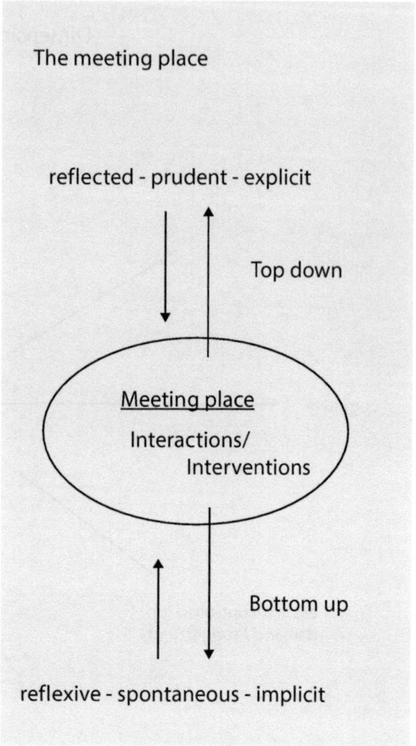

(Allen and Fonagy 2006). The pretend mode is predominant in the person concerned. The interlocutor often misses the reality and comprehensibility.

Especially traumatized people, patients with paranoid personality traits or borderline personality disorder often try to find out what the other person means, feels, thinks, believes or could do. They try to protect themselves from this even before it is obvious, often even before the other person even suspects what he or she is being accused of. This leads to over- and misinterpretations that are difficult to get out of the world (over-attribution). The problem is that "the genuine" often remains unrecognized or no consensus can be reached.

Abuse of Mentalizing

Abuse of mentalizing refers to mentalizing that appears above average at first glance, but which—and this is the insight at second glance—is used to manipulate others selfishly (Bateman and Fonagy 2006). This disorder is found in varying degrees and severity, for example, in people who are predominantly in the teleological mode, in antisocial and psychopathic patients, and in murderers. The disorder is characterized by a below-average level or even absence of emotional empathy and an unrestricted capacity for cognitive empathy (Blair 2005). Sometimes the lack of emotional empathy can be recognized by the fact that the other person often makes use of clichés to conceal the lack of empathy.

Table 3.1 Prototypical examples of mentalization profiles. (After Taubner 2015)

	Internal	External	Self	Other	Cognitive	Affective
Borderline personality disorder	Very low	Very high	Very low	Low	Very low	High
Narcissistic personality disorder	Average	Low	Average	Very low	Very high	Very low

3.4 Mentalizing in Psychotherapy as a Prerequisite for "Spirited" Change

In psychotherapy, the task now is to assess the patient's mentalizing ability. In outpatient practice, it is usually sufficient to imagine the mentalization star as a basis for a survey during the first interviews and to consider the different dimensions in one's own questions. In the inpatient context, a systematic structural diagnosis is usually carried out. At the same time, the mentalization profiles reveal which dimensions should be further promoted or developed. Examples of profiles and their potential for change and improvement are shown in Table 3.1.

For the topic of power/powerlessness, the mentalization dimensions relate specifically to the topics of

- Power/powerlessness of thought and emotion,
- Power/powerlessness of inner images and outer circumstances,
- Power/powerlessness of one's own self-reference and reference to others,
- Power/powerlessness of spontaneous reaction and controlled reflection (also through stimulation by others).

3.5 Mentalising Power/Powerlessness at the Different Levels

3.5.1 Power/Powerlessness in Contingency Experience and Difficulties with Affect Differentiation

All attacks have an immediate effect, are not filtered, cannot be reflected, are indeterminate, distinctions are not possible. It is a feeling of being absolutely at the mercy and not being able to react. In the positive case it is such that a concordant interplay triggers a great sense of well-being. The person feels powerful, momentarily also exerts himself and does not yet know that his experience depends on the matching reaction of the counterpart (contingent mirroring).

It is an experience that one must imagine as that of an infant up to the 3rd month of life. The infant experiences indeterminately, it does not yet know a no or cannot assign it. If the baby is mirrored appropriately or contingently by its parents, it feels good. Most of all it likes concordance.

Descriptions of patients in contingent experience, which only reflect what is observable and (in this situation) do not relate to teleological interpretations or intentional aspects, do not contain explanatory connections and always seem fragmented. As a psychotherapist it can be difficult to get an idea of the patient's everyday world.

► Example

Patient A witnessed a fight. He describes the situation: "The man was wearing a black sweater." (Neither teleological aspect nor motive) He describes the action: "The man was beating." (Neither teleological aspect nor motive for action) He describes a feeling, a thought, a statement "The woman was sad … She thought he was trying to help her." (The description is not completed by an explanation by means of a teleological aspect or mental states)

When asked by the psychotherapist about goal or purpose or motive, the response might be, "You're the expert. You must know that." ◄

3.5.2 Power/Powerlessness in the Targeted or Teleological Mode

A process is considered real when it can be observed or physically experienced. Having seen through cause and effect principles (at the level of physical reality) gives the person the feeling of having understood the world. He/she feels powerful when the world works. Principle is often: one must use the necessary means. Power struggle is accepted as a necessary evil. Regulation of powerlessness experience seems to be possible only by changes in external reality. Accordingly, the concern of another must be expressed through actions so that the person feels "seen". It is as if external evidence is always needed.

As a psychotherapist, it is easy to feel manipulated. Descriptions of patients in the targeted mode refer to observables, indicate teleological interpretations and do not contain motives.

► Example

Patient B describes the same brawl. He describes purposeful action. For example, he would say, "The man hit the woman to steal her money." (No motive for action)

When the psychotherapist asks about motives, the response might be, "I told you so." ◄

3.5.3 Power/Powerlessness in the Equivalence Mode

In the equivalence mode, inner and outer reality are equated, according to the motto: "As soon as I feel such and such, I must fear that it will also occur in reality according to my feeling. When this distinction is not made, feeling powerless becomes reality. Instead of saying 'I feel powerless', the person insists on saying 'I am powerless'. Instead of 'I feel worthless,' the thought 'I am worth nothing' arises." Threats have the same effect as completed actions. Thoughts and feelings can quickly have a devastating quality in the equivalence mode.

Conversely, successes can create a sense of grandiosity. Also, the claim that one knows what the other is thinking gives a conviction of superiority and power. Attributions seem immovable: "It's because of my mother that I don't have a chance in life."

As a psychotherapist, one is often afraid that something one has said will immediately turn into reality or conjure up disaster scenarios in the patient.

► Example

Patient C describes the same brawl. He is convinced that he has the correct interpretation. For example, he would say: "The man beat the woman to steal her money. He is quite a poor wretch; I saw that at once. He certainly didn't know how else to get money. That was an act of desperation."

When asked by the psychotherapist if there were other motives, "No, I'm sure of that. I hope he doesn't kill himself." ◄

3.5.4 Power/Powerlessness in the Pretend Mode

The pretend mode is characterized by endless conversations that have little relation to reality and that do not set any inner-psychic processes in motion. The one who is in this mode feels safe and powerful in insinuating and playing and creates impotent states of emptiness and meaninglessness in the other person. It seems like having a creative person in front of you, which the one can also be as a mercurial idea generator if you make yourself completely available and go along with every little game and let yourself be harnessed. Then the other person feels powerful, as if he/she alone, as the idea giver, has shaped and realized the creative process; but you yourself quickly feel rushed and powerless, because it is impossible to keep up with the pace of ever new ideas in realization. The as-if world is, in the positive, a fascinatingly powerful world of magic, enchantment, play; in the negative, a devouringly powerful world of pretences, acting, negation.

As a psychotherapist, one feels—after initial fascination—boredom because there is no depth, there seems to be no centre to talk about in more depth.

► Example

Patient D describes the same brawl. He plays with different interpretations. For example, he would say: "The man hit the woman, I don't know, could be to steal her money, but on the other hand, why should he? Who knows if she even had any money on her. Gee, if this keeps up. Maybe there'll be more. Well, I think the police should do more than that. I wonder if the woman is still in the hospital."

When the psychotherapist asked why the man had struck: "You hear so much. Maybe it was a relationship. I read the other day … " ◄

3.5.5 Power/Powerlessness in Reflective Mode: Meaning of Empathy and Caring

Descriptions that refer to observables and at the same time want to explain or struggle to explain why someone acts the way he/she does, indicate that someone is trying to explain someone else's behavior based on mental states. Power and powerlessness, as long as the patient can hold this mode, are understood in an intentional context. The patient includes mental states, e.g., motives, feelings, assumptions, intentions, presumptions, desires, hopes. Additionally, pretenses, needs, beliefs, planning can be considered. It becomes possible to put oneself in the perspective of other people and to see the world through their eyes. Along with this, the limited possibility of knowing exactly what the other person is thinking and feeling is also acknowledged. It is then explicitly clear that the same event can be seen from different perspectives and different points of view are possible. It is important to have empathy and sensitivity, and a conception of the complexity of mental states. There is an explicit recognition that everyone has limited power over their own and others' wishes, thoughts and desires in the real world. Notions of caring and responsibility to those weaker than oneself emerge.

All in all, there is the recognition of the temporal limitedness of a certain mental state and thus also implicitly of the corresponding behavior. This also makes a toleration of feelings of powerlessness possible in principle.

As a psychotherapist, you feel compassion, you are good at putting yourself in the patient's situation and point of view. The conversation can take place on a symbolic level; a look or a word is often enough for the patient to know that you care, have compassion or are conflicted.

► Example

Patient E describes the same brawl. He hints at empathy and caring. For example, he would say, "The man hit the woman; that must have been painful for her. There was a lot of bleeding. I don't know if they took her to the hospital right away. I certainly hope so. Usually, after all, they don't interrogate until they've received medical attention. The perpetrator had a deadpan expression. It seemed to me he wasn't sorry. Sometimes I wonder how come someone can be so cold. It kind of scares me."

When asked by the psychotherapist what scared him: "My father was actually a good man, but come to think of it, I was often afraid of him. It was never quite clear why, but sometimes he would yell out of nowhere. My mother said it was stressful for him at work then. But he never said that." ◄

In the reflective mode, one's own ethics and value system take on a high significance. These relativize a power/powerlessness thinking in the sense of an absolute above, below thinking that offers no lasting security. According to Arendt (1963), "power by its very nature is never capable of offering a substitute for the security and stability of actual reality" (ibid., p. 351).

In psychotherapy, it is essential to offer the patient security and stability in the actual relationship, to strengthen the patient's sense of power together with him, and to overcome his experience of powerlessness. Ten concrete steps are named as examples in each case:

Ten Steps to the Acquisition of Power Experience in Psychotherapy
Therapist and patient work on

1. the conviction that they can influence their own surroundings,
2. the notion of being able to influence others,
3. the ability to anticipate,
4. the ability to empathize with others,
5. the ability to deal with one's own feelings,
6. the ability to deal with your own thoughts,
7. the ability to form caring relationships,
8. the ability to negotiate,
9. the ability to separate yourself,
10. the ability to endure powerlessness and fear.

Ten Steps Against Powerlessness
Therapist and patient work on

1. the attitude that situations can be changed—together if necessary,
2. the ability not to flee, but to remain open and to perceive,
3. reflection on media and sources of information,
4. the willingness to discuss in therapy, in everyday life, with friends, relatives,
5. the attitude that our consumer behaviour can make a difference,
6. the capacity for solidarity,
7. the motivation to get involved for oneself and others,
8. the ability to develop new perspectives and possibilities,
9. the ability to act and cooperate with others and to dream,
10. the willingness to treat all people with empathy and care.

The following discusses how a psychotherapist can recognize constructive and destructive uses of power.

References

Allen JG, Fonagy P (2006) Mentalisierungsgestützte Therapie. Klett-Cotta, Stuttgart. 2009
Arendt H (1963) Wahrheit und Politik. In: Wahrheit und Lüge in der Politik. Zwei Essays. Piper, München 1972

Bateson G (1996) Ökologie des Geistes: anthropologische, psychologische, biologische und epistemologische Perspektiven. Suhrkamp, Frankfurt a.M
Blair RJR (2005) Responding to the emotions of others: Dissociating forms of empathy through the study of typical and psychiatric populations. Conscious Cognit 14:698–718
Böllinger L (2008) Macht. In: Mertens W, Waldvogel B (Hrsg) Handbuch psychoanalytischer Grundbegriffe. Kohlhammer, Stuttgart, S. 441–446
Fink-Eitel H (1992) Dialektik der Macht. In: Angehrn E et al. (Hrsg) Dialektischer Negativismus. Suhrkamp, Frankfurt a.M., S. 35–56
Fonagy P, Gergely G, Jurist E, Target M (2004) Affektregulierung, Mentalisierung und die Entwicklung des Selbst. Klett-Cotta, Stuttgart
Foucault M (1987) Das Subjekt und die Macht. In: Hubert L, Dreyfus PR (eds) Michel Foucault. Jenseits von Strukturalismus und Hermeneutik. Athenäum, Frankfurt a.M., pp 241–261
Grof S (1975) Topographie des Unbewussten: LSD im Dienst der tiefenpsychologischen Forschung. Klett-Cotta, Stuttgart
Gruen A (1984) Der Verrat am Selbst. Die Angst vor Autonomie bei Mann und Frau. Causa, München
Gruen A (2016) Wider die kalte Vernunft. Klett-Cotta, Stuttgart
Habermas J (1981) Philosophisch-politische Profile. Suhrkamp, Frankfurt a.M
Habermas J (1985) Die neue Unübersichtlichkeit. Kleine Politische Schriften V. Suhrkamp, Frankfurt a.M
Häusel HG (2008) Brain view. Haufe, Planegg
Hesse H (1987) Demian. GW Bd. 5. Suhrkamp, Frankfurt a.M.
Janov A (1981) Gefangen im Schmerz. Fischer, Frankfurt a.M
Janov A (1993) Der neue Urschrei: Fortschritt in der Primärtherapie. Fischer, Frankfurt a.M
Janov A (2000) The biology of love. Prometheus, New York
Janov A (2007) Die Janov-Lösung. Primärtherapie—Ein Weg aus der Depression. SterlinHouse Books, Pittsburgh
Jurist EL (2008) Mind and yours. In: Jurist EL, Slade A, Bergner S (eds) Mind to mind. Infant research, neuroscience and psychoanalysis. Other Press, New York
Kraus B (2002) Konstruktivismus—Kommunikation—Soziale Arbeit. Radikalkonstruktivistische Betrachtungen zu den Bedingungen des sozialpädagogischen Interaktionsverhältnisses. Carl-Auer-Systeme, Heidelberg
Luhmann N (1975) Macht, 4. Aufl. UTB, Stuttgart. 2012
Luyten P, Fonagy P, Lowyck B, Vermote R (2011) Assessment of mentalization. In: Bateman AW, Fonagy P (eds) Handbook of mentalizing in mental health practice. American Psychiatric Pub., Washington, DC, pp 43–65
Machiavelli N (1513) Il Principe. Übs. und hrsg. von Rudolf Zorn. Kröner, Stuttgart. 1972
Miller A (1979) Das Drama des begabten Kindes. Suhrkamp, Berlin
Miller A (2007) Dein gerettetes Leben. Suhrkamp, Berlin
Nietzsche F (1980) Sämtliche Werke. Kritische Studienausgabe in 15 Bänden, 3. Aufl. Hrsg. von Giorgio Colli und Mazzino Montinari. dtv, München 2009
Panksepp J (2003) Feeling the pain of social loss. Science 302:237–239
Portele G (1989) Autonomie, Macht, Liebe. Konsequenzen der Selbstreferentialität. Suhrkamp, Frankfurt a.M.
Portele G, Roessler K (1994) Macht und Psychotherapie. Ein Dialog. Edition Humanistische Psychologie, Köln
Rank O (1924) Das Trauma der Geburt und seine Bedeutung für die Psychoanalyse. Psychosozial-Verlag, Gießen. 2007
Roth G, Strüber N (2014) Wie das Gehirn die Seele macht. Klett-Cotta, Stuttgart
Sapute AB, Lieberman MD (2006) Integrating automatic and controlled processes into neurocognitive models of social cognition. Brain Res 1079(1):86–97
Schore AN (1994) Affect regulation and the origin of the self. Lawrence Erlbaum, Hillsdale, NJ
Schultz-Venrath U (2013) Lehrbuch Mentalisieren. Klett-Cotta, Stuttgart
Taubner S (2015) Konzept Mentalisieren. Psychosozial-Verlag, Gießen
Upledger JE (1996) Auf den inneren Arzt hören. Hugendubel, München

Weber M (1922) Wirtschaft und Gesellschaft. Siebeck, Tübingen
Weiss J (1993) How Psychotherapy Works. Guilford Press, New York
Winnicott DW (1965) Reifungsprozesse und fördernde Umwelt. Studien zur Theorie der emotionalen Entwicklung. Gießen, Psychosozial-Verlag, p 2002
Willi J (1975) Die Zweierbeziehung. Spannungsursachen, Störungsmuster, Klärungsprozesse, Lösungsmodelle. Rowohlt, Reinbek bei Hamburg

As a Psychotherapist, How Do I Recognize Constructive and Destructive Use of Power?

Contents

M.-L. Althoff, *Mentalizing Power and Powerlessness*,
https://doi.org/10.1007/978-3-662-66119-2_4

It is crucial for the success of psychotherapy to be able to distinguish between the constructive and destructive use of power. The guiding question of this chapter is which types and forms of expression of constructive and destructive exercise of power can be found on the part of psychotherapists and patients. In this context, it will also be outlined how powerlessness can manifest itself on both sides. Finally, the constructive and destructive influence of the system (mostly as a background context) is discussed.

"The Socratic 'It is better to suffer injustice than to do injustice' is a statement and not a commandment, and it is a statement that makes a truth claim and is therefore not an opinion" (Arendt 1963a, p. 343). Hannah Arendt raises the question whether this statement by Socrates does not contradict the conviction that the validity of philosophical truths cannot be proven. The claim of validity stemmed from the fact that Socrates staked his life on it. He refused to evade the execution of the death sentence. "The sentence did Socrates wrong, but it was legally incontestable; to evade it would have been to do wrong" (ibid.). Arendt agrees with Nietzsche who writes, "I make of a philosopher just so much as he is able to make an example" (Nietzsche 1874). I will follow this principle in my book, i.e., where I think my thoughts may not be immediately obvious, I will prove them by practice. Empiricism may like to follow casuistry. "Thus we make clear what courage is by thinking of Achill, and we shall think of Jesus of Nazareth or of St. Francis if we want to know what goodness is. The examples teach or persuade by inspiration, so that it seems to us that we are imitating—the 'imitatio Christi' for example—we are behaving according to an example whenever we behave in terms of a moral principle." (Arendt 1963a, p. 343)

If we start from the original meaning of the word, then the Latin means

- **struere to** build, to layer, to pile up, to erect, to stack, to lay one on top of the other, side by side, to pile up. It is about recognizing and building structure in its layering, also the term formation "psychic structure" leans on this word. **strueris** means "you are being built". Already the activities—in a figurative sense—building psychic structure, assembling I understand as constructive exercise of power.
- **construere** also means to build, but more in the sense of to build, to erect, to pile together. Here it tends to be more about the realization of a building plan. Something is being built, constructed. **construeris** also means "you are being built".
- **destruere** means to destroy, to tear down. Something that stands and has been created is destroyed. **destrueris** means "you will be destroyed".

Both are part of life: Building up and tearing down, the constructive and the destructive. Both belong to our wealth of experience.

There are things which are built and which we enjoy. But there are also things that are built and seem questionable to us, e.g. the tallest building in the world, one-sided competition, missile defence systems. In this respect, building is in itself neutral, neither good nor bad. By constructive exercise of power in psychotherapy I mean an exercise of power that is morally judged to be good, that is supported by ethical-moral principles and is directed towards a goal that is accepted by the patient and the psychotherapist (▶ Sect. 4.1).

There are things that are destroyed, and (almost) everyone agrees, e.g. the demolition of a dilapidated or asbestos-contaminated building that represents a danger, the abolition of authoritarian-violent systems, the displacement of old structures of antiquated psychiatry, psychotherapy and pedagogy, the paralysis of a perverted part of the personality, the destruction of certain illusions. Destructive in the narrower, evaluative sense is what I will call in the following text an exercise of power that aims at destruction for the sake of destruction out of lower ego-like motives and by using also dubious means (▶ Sect. 4.2).

The perceived or actual power of psychotherapists makes some potential patients shy away from therapy. What is the source of power in a concrete therapeutic situation? How is it that one person believes he or she has more power than another? Sometimes psychotherapists also perceive certain patients as very powerful. If one wants to master such a relationship constellation, even in the case of conflict-laden topics, one cannot avoid the topic of power. First of all, one should think about from which **sources** one can mobilize which power when needed. From these thoughts a reflective and constructive handling of power can develop and the danger of abuse of power can be prevented.

4.1 Personality

If one wants to exercise power, one must be able to inflict positive or negative things on another, even against the other's reluctance (Max Weber). Furthermore, one must be seen as someone who not only can, but will do so if necessary. If one is not trusted with the necessary toughness or determination, one loses respect and credibility in the eyes of the other. This is where the difficulties of exercising power by harmony-seeking and good-natured people already begin.

Managers, for example, are expected to be able to carry out announced (and also unannounced) measures or sanctions, e.g. to confront employees who do not apply themselves sufficiently, to terminate constant complainers and worriers and to praise and promote committed colleagues (▶ Chap. 2). This determination, straightforwardness, ability to make decisions, and certainly willingness to engage in conflict—all communicate to the other, but are by no means to be equated with an authoritarian demeanor. There is no typical power style, no typical appearance. People appear differently depending on their field of life or profession, on their age, on their gender. Think of well-known and influential politicians, actors, scientists, psychotherapists! As everywhere, what counts in the end is neither a masquerade nor words alone, but deeds done with a noticeable determination.

4.2 Status and Role

The power associated with a role or status derives from the fact that it is inherent in a particular office or position. It is conferred upon the incumbent with that position. This gives him or her certain possibilities or powers which, conversely, subordinates do not have towards him or her.

The psychotherapist obtains this status with the healing licence granted by law.

(a) If there is a basis of trust in psychotherapy, then the patient opens up unilaterally—i.e. without the alternating self-opening of the therapist—with many parts of his self, e.g. also with strongly shame-ridden ones. If this is not handled carefully, unbearable feelings of shame and mortification can be the result. The patient rightly fears this power of the psychotherapist and forms resistance.

(b) But this does not mean that the patient is always automatically powerless or helpless. In psychotherapy, as a psychotherapist, you do have the role of provider. But one is also dependent on the patient. You can feel this dependence more acutely the more you assess the patient as likely to complain or speak ill of you to the health insurance company or the board, or as likely to have sadistic traits. It becomes especially critical when the patient's willingness to go to higher authorities or to torment others coincides with the psychotherapist's lack of defensibility. Some patients unconsciously take advantage of this, behaving, for example, aggressively and unpredictably or helplessly and ill. They try to force the psychotherapist to do things he did not want to do. The aggressive variety is potentially intimidating; the helpless variety of exercising power, called the power of weakness, is at least as difficult to deal with as the aggressive pressure. Both can leave the psychotherapist feeling not only low on power, but helpless and powerless.

(c) If the patient, who feels powerless and helpless, complains with high suffering pressure, one gets under pressure. Many patients tread water in therapy over a period of time and retain the same difficulties despite having gained insight in the meantime. Then neither of them feels powerful.

As a psychotherapist, one should always be aware that the power of position or status is also a granted power that can be taken away from one moment to the next. Consider, for example, that one can be suspected of having committed a criminal act and, although innocent, may not be able to credibly refute it.

As a psychotherapist, one is given different powers in different roles, e.g. as a practitioner, supervisor, reviewer, examiner, lecturer, professional representative. The same applies, incidentally, to staff in a psychotherapeutic practice who report to the practice owner. This power is often greater than is commensurate with formal status. It is a matter of decision-making power, but it is always of an advocacy, suggestion nature. One does not have a formal decision-making power towards the commissioning people or institutions, and the decision-making power can be withdrawn at any time. That one usually nevertheless feels and, in the perception of others, possesses power and influence is partly because one may have an impressive personality, partly because of knowledge of supportive relationships, but one also feels the conferred power that is unspokenly associated with the assignment of a particular function or task.

This has its pitfalls: One may be granted a lot of power from one moment to the next and may not be able to handle it responsibly enough. It may be that one then consciously does not accept this power or unconsciously does not like to recognize it and then a large part of one's own creative possibilities remains unused. What is more difficult is when one relates this increase in power to oneself personally and uses it in an egocentric and self-important manner, which may ultimately amount to mild or severe forms of abuse of power. Moreover, granted power is always a power dependent on others, since it can—at least theoretically—be withdrawn at any time. Absolute power exists, in my opinion, only as freedom, and that is when one is always aware of one's decision-making possibilities, in the sense formulated by Nietzsche of the "will to power" or the "will to one's own destiny." The power bestowed is valid only as long as the principal stands firmly by his mandate. Even at the first signals of motivation to change or restructure shown by the principal, the power conferred wavers considerably. Current examples of this are the periodic tendencies to break up the associations of doctors, to replace the peer review process, to change the structure of psychotherapeutic training, to reform the Psychotherapists Act, to recognize new psychotherapeutic procedures or not, to name but a few. In response to such signals, some people withdraw preventively, reposition themselves, get into crises of meaning and lose joy, confidence and commitment.

4.3 Knowledge of Institutions, Laws and Relationships

Knowledge of how the institutions involved function, which laws govern them, and which professional and private relationships are fundamental can confer factual or perceived power, and it complements the factors of personality and status.

This knowledge, on the part of the psychotherapist, refers to how sure one is of knowing the institutional, status and legal regulations and proposals, as well as one's own relationships, and thus having the power to be able to comply with them (or to deliberately ignore them) or to be able to rely on them. It also refers to being clear about how far one's influence extends. In one's own practice or practice space, one may sometimes feel like an isolated lone wolf, but it can be helpful (and is also part of the necessary knowledge of a psychotherapist) to be aware of which helpers (e.g. police, ambulance, youth welfare office) one can mobilise and which people (e.g. colleagues, supervisors, family members, friends) one can count on for support when needed. One could now think that it is about how big one's own "house power" is. However, that is not what I have in mind here. For me it is about how confident and influential one feels with this knowledge to be able to advise the patient well about therapeutic options and to make a competent and committed impression. For some therapists, depending on their power and personality type, this may go so far as to adopt a paternalistic attitude, that is, an attitude of well-meaning paternal authority.

As a patient, you can compensate for an inferior position in comparison to the psychotherapist by fully informing yourself about your rights as a patient and the conditions of reimbursement by the health insurance company, as well as reflecting on the therapist's idiosyncrasies and attitudes, and by asking friends and family for advice. In this way, one can then also better judge how comprehensively the psychotherapist informs one. Sometimes one may feel so confident that one trusts the psychotherapist completely. Sometimes one will sense the feeling or the urge to take action oneself in order to build up a protection against one's own good faith being severely disappointed and leading to a feeling of powerlessness.

It becomes clear that the source of power knowledge of institutions, laws and relationships is linked to the sources of personality and status. Status and relationships also interact; consider, for example, a situation in which preferential support is given to someone whom you judge to be influential or whose referrer you judge to be important or from whom you hope to benefit. Related to the personality of the psychotherapist and also that of the patient is the knowledge of relationships that results from whether or how far you trust the other person, but also what you trust them to do. And it goes beyond both parties involved, because trust also depends on what relationships, with other people or institutions, you have been able to build up in your life, whether there are people or institutions who feel committed to yourself and who support you, and what hopes and fears others associate with you.

If you want to realize constructive and conscious power management, the first thing you should do is develop an interest in this subject. By buying or borrowing this book, this has already happened. Step two is fundamentally about expanding your own ability to deal with conflict and to endure tension, unresolved issues and disharmony, and about building and maintaining a relationship with your counterpart. One should be able to endure being perceived as friendly-helpful at times and strict-unyielding at others, without immediately having to justify oneself or retreat. For this, for example, the role of "Everybody's Darling" must be overcome. Of course, the shift between the two should not be guided by whims, but by feelings and considerations appropriate to the situation. It seems to me important to cultivate one's relationship to power. This involves making an effort to learn about destructive and self-centered traits, as well as conflict-avoidance tendencies, such as are present in each of us, in oneself and, if possible, to reduce them. And it is part of this to look for places of reflection with others (e.g. intervision, supervision) in addition to one's own reflection. I will now first deal with the forms of constructive exercise of power and then with the forms of destructive exercise of power.

4.4 Constructive Use of Power in Psychotherapy

To master the constructive exercise of power in word and deed requires—unless one is a natural in this field—some practice. Many are already afraid of the peaceful forms of power. Their need for harmony often gets in the way. They are unable to fight, let alone actively escalate the situation, and give up before they reach their goal. Possibly they are then (unconsciously) also afraid of a disappointment or overreaction and protect themselves from it. Still others always have to start from 0 to 100 and explode, scream, say things they regret afterwards. Here are a few suggestions on how constructive exercise of power can look like or succeed.

Fritz Künkel, known as an individual psychologist and colleague of Alfred Adler, with whom there was later a break, said that the effect of power (constructive or destructive) depends on whether the power is used "unbiased" or "ego-like" (cf. Künkel 1929, 1935). Someone who learns to be unbiased will be able to put his or her ego in the service of a cause and feel it in the dedication to supra-personal goals and values or community-promoting developments, projects, ideas. According to Künkel, impartiality is therefore not to be equated with emotional coldness and sobriety, but rather to be understood in the meaning of "appropriate", so that one can say, for example, that impartiality in a particular situation is composed of kindness, care, understanding and empathy for the other. Egocentricity, on the other hand, according to Künkel, means having a fear of life and of one's fellow human beings, self-preservation, loneliness and an excessive striving for security, and directing one's intentions against the community. This happens when power is used e.g. self-centredly, only to put oneself above others, to make others small, to destroy. Depending on the predominance of the unbiased or the egocentricity, the communication of a person with the environment is shaped. According to Künkel, egocentricity is combined with irritability, impartiality with sensitivity. The irritable person gets into permanent conflicts with his environment, the sensitive person can differentiate and sense the mental state of others and derive an understanding for himself and others from this (ibid.). In the following, I would like to use the distinction "unbiased" and "ego-like".

The environment senses this difference immediately and reacts accordingly. Constructive, i.e. unbiased, exercise of power is often hardly noticeable or is perceived as a beneficial, orderly activity. It has the goal of setting the course, stimulating perspectives and mobilizing energies.

The ego-like exercise of power, on the other hand, makes itself immediately felt through the noticeable devaluation and degradation, as the person is concerned with wanting to establish their own superiority through slights and humiliations. Some react consciously or unconsciously by going into the role of the victim, others go into the silent suffering or mortification, still others immediately leave the relationship or identify with this kind of exercise of power, i.e. with the aggressor.

4.4.1 Constructive Exercise of Power By the Patient

What does constructive exercise of power on the part of the patient look like in concrete terms? I structure the answer—without claiming completeness—along the subdivision of personality, status and knowledge. Children with a normal development of mentalization are able to use these constructive forms of exercising power from the age of 4 or 5. If they have not reached this level of mentalization, one can almost certainly observe either aggressive and destructive power behavior or exaggerated obedience and docility.

- **Personality**

For example, the patient—regardless of age—must bring with him/her an ability for therapeutic ego splitting (Sterba 1934) that is sufficient for the planned therapy, i.e. the ability to split the ego into an observing and an experiencing part. If the patient brings this ability into the joint work, he/she implicitly expects a similar response from the therapist.

Another form of the constructive exercise of power by patients is that in phases in which they idealise the psychotherapist "Now I am in therapy with you; now everything will be all right", they exercise power by demanding a reaction from the therapist. A reaction is also demanded when patients take the view that the psychotherapist as a human being does not know everything either and is not perfect.

Psychotherapists also sense the exercise of power by patients when they ask for realistic goal perspectives. Patients exercise constructive power when they challenge their psychotherapists to discuss goals and expectations. Patients challenge psychotherapists when they want to engage in dialogue about procedure and method. They exert gentle pressure when they formulate high expectations of honesty and truthfulness.

Patients often formulate emphatically that they finally need someone who can understand them. They formulate their suffering and the need for change very emphatically. They declare themselves ready for negotiations about frequency, times, holiday arrangements and other framework components. They exercise power indirectly when they admit to the psychotherapist that they themselves are despondent and think he/she knows what to do. They sometimes take the lead when they go into regression. The psychotherapist has to react or intervene in a controlling way. They resist the therapist's rapid action.

■ Status

In its quietest form, a criterion for the presence of power, being coerced, is not felt by the psychotherapist. The patient grants the psychotherapist cooperation because the psychotherapist is held in high esteem, because he/she will be dependent on his/her support and because he/she wants to secure his/her goodwill – according to the motto "I give so that you give". If one doubts that this mutual giving and taking has something to do with power, then one should always test (in one's mind) the "counter test". Would you give the same reliability and support to another stranger if they had less competence and influence? If you answer in the negative, then cooperation has something to do with the patient's power.

Power lives from cooperation. If the exerciser of power does not want to use force, he/she is dependent on the concession of the counterpart. It is extremely rare that a patient wants to directly force a psychotherapist to treat him/her. He/she knows that it pays to get the therapist's consent through persuasion and negotiation.

■ Knowledge

Patients can inform themselves about the possibilities of therapy financed by the health insurance fund, about institutions such as the medical or psychotherapeutic associations and laws, e.g. on patients' rights and the provision fee. They can also find out about the psychotherapeutic procedure offered by the psychotherapist and reflect on their own goals and wishes. They can consider who in their environment can answer questions about psychotherapy.

Patients, too, know consciously or unconsciously that power is always maintained in roughly equal parts by those who submit and by those who exercise it. Because some play along, others have the power. As a psychotherapist, for example, you sense this the moment a patient fails to show up without a cancellation. Even if others think primarily of the abuse of power when they think of power, for example, of the cheating of advantages, unscrupulous machinations, suppression of freedom of opinion, etc., it is necessary precisely then to make it clear with determination that one can make use of constructive power in order to drive forward processes of change that are necessary in the interest of achieving the goal. It is often the case that without the willingness to use power—if at all—profound changes cannot be realised in the time available (imperative of necessity, expediency and economic efficiency of psychotherapy financed by the health insurance system).

Kraus (2013, p. 126) distinguishes between instructive and destructive power. For him, instructive means taking the chance to "determine the behaviour and thinking of another". Destructive means perceiving the chance to "reduce the possibilities of another". I think it is still within the realm of constructive exercise of power to "reduce the possibilities of another". Destructive exercise of power, in my opinion, only begins where the end justifies the means and unfair or violent methods are used.

If, as an alternative to exercising power, one **always** remains on a negotiating standpoint, it often comes down to the "lowest common denominator" or a "lazy compromise" or a "half-hearted solution", of which one is no longer convinced oneself. So if you as a psychotherapist do not want to choose this alternative, you also need **the courage of power**.

4.4.2 Constructive Exercise of Power By the Psychotherapist

In this process, enforcement in the sense of setting the course, activating resources and persuasion usually takes place almost inconspicuously, so that untrained observers hardly notice the use of power. Compromises can initially still be fragile and marked by some silent reservations. Thinking power-consciously means recognizing these reservations, even without voicing them, and trying to resolve them through communication, involvement, and by making demands, i.e., asking for one's own contributions. Thinking in terms of power also means being aware that once a goal has been agreed upon, it has not yet been achieved and that it makes sense to ensure tangible results at an early stage, and to make it clear time and again that one is still firmly committed to the goal or project. Here, too, the exercise of power has nothing to do with fighting, but is demonstrated by the intelligent shaping of processes and the early setting of signals, which even means conflict prevention.

Here, too, observers usually do not even notice that power has been exercised because it happens so "bloodlessly" and without conflict. The people concerned, however, sense the unconditional determination behind the "soft surface". This friendliness and commitment, however, is not a mask, as it is sometimes misunderstood, a cloak that is supposed to cover up the iron hardness lying behind it, but friendliness and commitment are the expression of a basic attitude that does not aim at defeating and suppressing, but at shaping through bringing together, orientation and integration.

Of course, even the gentlest exercise of power does not always please those affected; sometimes they react to the forced change of course with more or less pronounced displeasure. You have to be able to live with this at times if you see power as a necessary instrument for achieving goals and consequently also use it as an opportunity to shape things. Of course, it is always more pleasant when conviction, rather than gentle coercion, leads to the goal, but the reality is that not every counterpart can be convinced immediately because, for example, fears, reservations or ignorance stand in the way. In such a case—as already mentioned—the only option is the time-consuming search for a compromise, the abandonment of the project or the **courage to use power**.

What does constructive exercise of power on the part of the psychotherapist look like in concrete terms? Again, I structure the answer along the domains of personality, status and knowledge.

▪ Personality

Psychotherapists—just like patients—need the ability for therapeutic ego splitting (Sterba 1934), i.e. the ability to split the ego into an observing and reflecting part and an experiencing part. You must expect this ability from yourself and must also be able to make it clear to the patient that this ability is expected of him or her. The observing part analyzes the issues, questions, and structures interventions; the experiencing part is compassionate, empathic, and relates emotionally. This does not mean, however, to adopt a cold and distanced stance overall, but to take the different points of view and emotional constitutions in the therapeutic encounter alternately oneself and to weigh them against each other.

Furthermore, in order to exercise power constructively, psychotherapists need the ability to demand and maintain a working alliance (Greenson 1967) as part of the interactional process, even in the face of resistance.

They need the ability to use peaceful forms of power. Peaceful forms include e.g. the competences to persuade, to argue, to negotiate, to make offers, to make compromises. Being too peaceful means not being able to enforce even the simplest things.

It can become necessary, if peaceful forms are of no avail, that the option of a fighting side comes into play. The question then arises as to how a struggle should be conducted. How does one assert oneself or how does one defend oneself? As a psychotherapist, you now have to have an assessment of who you are dealing with. You have to know which playing field you are entering. Figuratively speaking: When you enter a fighting arena, you also have to expect that either the other person or you will get hurt. So you have to be aware of the risks, and you also have to have defined for yourself ethical boundaries of what is fair and how far you want to go.

In this respect, as a psychotherapist one should be clear about which instruments and weapons—figuratively speaking—one possesses and which may be used when. The more effective an instrument, the greater the potential danger it poses. A sword is more dangerous than a kitchen knife, a steamroller more dangerous than a rolling pin, an electric hedge trimmer more dangerous than a pair of nail scissors. But the dangers do not come from the devices and tools, but from when and how people bring them into use. And then, for example, even the rolling pin can be deadly. People with their morals, intentions and goals are decisive.

Being aware of one's personal power competence and one's power instruments also leads to an economy of power, because one does not wear oneself out so much, has more action alternatives available and can initiate actions in a more targeted manner.

▪ Status

Psychotherapists can use their competence to exert influence. The status allows and also provides a certain goal orientation. In addition, psychotherapists can use their expertise in concrete psychotherapeutic situations, e.g. in the form of psychoeducation. They can use the creative leeway offered by the status, e.g. make recommendations or initiate multimodal treatment options.

▪ Knowledge

As a psychotherapist, one can decide whether one feels more comfortable in practice as a lone wolf or in a community. Irrespective of this, it is important to know which institutions can provide assistance or support if necessary, in order to be able to act powerfully. The medical or psychotherapeutic associations, for example, offer advice to members and advice on professional law.

If one wants to make full use of one's own creative scope as a psychotherapist, one must be informed about legal and professional policy regulations and changes. Conversely, information deficits in the form of uncertainties can have a damaging effect on the therapeutic relationship.

It is also decisive which professional-political or scientific groups one joins. This determines how well one is oriented towards the latest state of information, discussion and theory and in which direction one is developing.

Where power is involved, one is (more or less often) manifestly or unconsciously concerned with powerlessness and helplessness, both as a patient and as a psychotherapist:

> Just as the demonstration of one's own powerlessness conceals one's own power, a demonstration of power compensates for one's own feelings of powerlessness. As a rule, we perceive the power of the other party, i.e., we deny it in ourselves and project it onto a counterpart. But power exists only as a relational phenomenon, i.e., power and powerlessness are two sides of a holistic phenomenon and are divided between the relational partners in the experience. A feeling of power would not be felt at all without a feeling of powerlessness experienced at the same time in the background. (Moeller 1982, p. 91)

Dealing constructively with the experience of powerlessness means, e.g., powerlessness

- to want to overcome without going into dominance,
- without falling into self-denial and self-harm,
- to be able to endure without having to shut off feelings and turn off thoughts,
- without getting into a destructive power struggle,

- to be able to disagree without considering one's own opinion as the only valid one,
- in a healthy way, i.e. without going into symptoms.

4.4.3 Constructive Exercise of Power By the System

In every psychotherapy there is always the influence of

- Association of Statutory Health Insurance as an organ of self-administration,
- Aid agencies,
- Private insurance,
- statutory health insurance funds,
- Psychotherapists' or doctors' associations as professional representative bodies with further training courses and pension schemes,
- democratic framework with Civil Code and Social Code as well as regulations on quality management (e.g. DIN ISO 9001),
- the framework of the psychotherapy guidelines with expert procedures for quality assurance and protection against recourse claims,
- Organisations and associations on the psychotherapist and patient side, such as patient representation in the Federal Joint Committee or the German Foundation for Patient Protection,
- Guidelines for the diagnosis and treatment of mental disorders,
- scientific standards of the procedures.

When these institutions or organizations play a role as power-exerting instances in the context of psychotherapy, this can happen in quite different ways. Psychotherapists and patients can refer to the power of laws and regulations and sometimes also "hide" behind them if they themselves do not want to personally represent and negotiate certain restrictions and limitations, e.g. the end of therapy. Then, in the perception of patient and psychotherapist, e.g. the Association of Statutory Health Insurance or the legislator of the psychotherapy guidelines or the reviewer exercises the power. However, psychotherapists and patients can also refer to laws and regulations, for example, if this expresses consideration for influential people whom one does not want to snub or with whom one does not want to make trouble. Both psychotherapists and patients refer to laws and regulations if they are sure that otherwise transgressions or misconduct, e.g. in the case of false statements in health examinations, can be admonished or, on the part of the psychotherapist, even punished, e.g. with withdrawal of the licence to practise.

Most of the time, both sides hesitate when they realize that a certain proposal is beyond their power and that they probably cannot enforce this way. A fortiori, they behave lawfully when it is in line with their ethics to want to comply with laws and regulations.

Of course, the power of the system is also respected when both sides fear damaging their own reputation by taking too radical a path. Moreover, they lose courage and shy away from disadvantages when psychotherapists or patients become fearful at the thought of possible resistance or counter-reactions from the system. This happens regardless of whether "unbiased" or "ego" motives are involved. They usually know that even beyond personal fear, pusillanimity and over-cautiousness, there are good reasons to consider not only the technical side of decisions, but also their "political dimension".

Three Aspects of the Constructive Power-political Dimension

▪ Cooperation and Good Relations

4

If one understands how power-political action works, one will no longer associate power only with the "power of those up there", but will know that everyone, including the powerful, is dependent on cooperation (▶ Chap. 2: Machiavelli sees power, among other things, as a revolutionary possibility).

Attention to the "political dimension" in planned projects is necessary because even board members, managing directors and administrators by no means have unlimited power. In order to be able to lead successfully, the leaders are also and especially dependent on the people they lead following them and behaving cooperatively. This does not mean that those led have to be enthusiastic about it, but they should be able to "live with it", i.e. the path taken must neither be questionable in terms of the matter at hand, nor must it have too much of a negative effect on the personal interests of those involved; in short, it must remain below the threshold that would cause those led to become indignant and show solidarity.

For purely power-political reasons, every functionary should only announce or commit himself to projects whose implementation he can also vouch for. Conversely, this means that he should refrain from projects that exceed his own real power.

To the same extent that power increases with a hierarchical position, so do dependencies, upwards, downwards and laterally.

▶ Example

Psychotherapy peer reviewers, for example, have a certain position of power with regard to the endorsement or non-endorsement of requested psychotherapy services. However, they are dependent on "above", have to adhere to the guidelines and are directly dependent on regulations issued by government and health insurers. They are dependent "downwards", i.e. psychotherapists can lodge an objection, complain to their association or the government. And they are "laterally" dependent on each other, because the group of experts discusses certain interpretations of the guidelines and tries to reach a consensus. For directors of training institutes for psychotherapy, these dependencies in all directions can be easily understood in a similar way. ◀

A project manager, an institute director, a board of directors or managing director is dependent on his salaried and freelance staff to implement the decisions made and projects announced in his interests and on the psychotherapists with a licence to practise or in training to accept them. It also makes an enormous difference whether the employees are committed and fully convinced to implement the decisions of their boss or whether they are half-hearted in their work.

It is even more difficult for political functionaries to enforce their own ideas on the psychotherapeutic profession. They are not subordinate to them and cannot be fired, as is the case with employees. They are members who vote. Their constructive input can only be gained. The members don't have to do anything they don't want to do. You even have to make it as easy as possible for them to vote.

These power relations and dependencies give rise to considerations in everyday actions that are part of so-called political behaviour. However, this is by no means an action that is dubiously or even disreputably motivated, but a highly reasonable behaviour. Anyone who plans for the long term as a board member, executive director, leader must consider the impact of their actions on their colleagues, officers, employees and members. It would be highly unwise to try to push through proposals for change without coordination and networking processes, thereby angering many and incurring even more scepticism and mistrust in future projects.

In political and professional networks, the rule is not to hurt each other, but to support each other. In order not to damage their network, the functionaries will, for reasons of common sense, think twice before taking a path that surprises the network partners and, in addition, has a negative impact on them. This is often criticised as "wangling", but from the point of view of those involved it is a necessary and sensible course of action.

■ Constructive Active Power Politics

How can we nevertheless succeed in advancing change projects, winning the necessary support for them and keeping resistance to a minimum from the outset? This requires active power politics in the sense of a systematic coordination of the promoters of this project. It must be considered which persons and organisations are affected in their concerns and interests by the desired changes and what influence they could have on any decisions and their implementation. It is then necessary to involve them so that a sufficient number of employees support the desired changes. Active power politics is then by no means to be equated with ruthless enforcement, but means above all the building of acceptance and support. At best, the principle applies to become active before others do, and to form alliances for something (unbiased) and not against someone (egoistic). Of course, it is always taken into account who is sent ahead to address whom. Being approached by a president, board of directors, important functionary or leader usually increases the prospects of a positive response. From the point of view of power politics, it often seems more effective to support someone who, because of his influence, can also help the other way round on a later occasion.

So cultivating communication and active contacts is an essential part of active power politics. At least as important, however, are substantive discussions and the pacification of conflicts of interest. This again requires communication, because—as already mentioned—allies should not be surprised by developments that are negative for them, because then trust can turn into mistrust and bitter antagonism, all the way to refusal of support and even revenge.

■ Acceptance and Support

In such a large support network, as it has been built up in the field of psychotherapy in recent decades, the persons involved are involved in innumerable communication contexts, and the most diverse forces try to exert influence on them.

Agreements and supportive pledges must be regularly renewed and reaffirmed, otherwise they lose their validity in the great play of forces. Conversely, this can also apply to opponents and critics, with whom a discussion should also be sought from time to time, so as not to contribute to a hardening of the fronts, but also to find out whether and, if so, how their opinion has changed or can be influenced.

The chances of gaining support for relevant (pertinent) projects by talking to the powerful and authoritative players are often not bad. Both managers and employees tend to say yes rather than no when in doubt when asked for support, especially when asked by influential people with whom they want to be on good terms. Of course, the contribution they are asked to make also plays a role in agreeing to support. Is it a matter of accepting a project that does not significantly affect their interests, or does it require greater commitment or even changes of their own? In the first case, a commitment is more likely.

4.5 Destructive Exercise of Power in Psychotherapy

Power has generally become a taboo subject, although it plays a role in all areas of our lives. Hardly anyone speaks openly about their own quest for power. This disturbed relationship to power has far-reaching consequences. For, of course, the significance of a topic does not disappear through its tabooing and non-observance. It merely escapes conscious control and professional access, and the result can be what fearful tabooing sought to avoid: uncontrolled, unrestrained, and abusive power. Tabooing has the effect that reflection on the subject is omitted, with the consequence that the handling of power remains unprofessional, arises from reflexes and not from a formative strategy of action, and that violent feelings of powerlessness remain unprocessed and often unconscious.

Being able to exercise power sometimes also means being able to force people to do something. In this context, "coercing" stands both for the threat of disadvantages and, if necessary, the carrying out of this threat, as well as for the promise of possible advantages. The exercise of power is also present where the threat or promise is unspoken and the exerciser of power tacitly relies on the imagination, i.e. on the fears and hopes of those whom he wishes to influence. Here the line between still constructive and already destructive exercise of power becomes very narrow.

It is sometimes difficult to recognize that destructive expressions of power already begin when, for example, someone starts a fight without having consciously intended to do so. For example, the repeated questions "Did you really think about it?" or "Did you really mean it?" can come across as threats or battle announcements. Then the person does not have to be surprised if the other person reacts with a counterattack. Destructive is also experienced when someone takes advantage of good faith. People are highly annoyed when they think their counterpart is cooperative and see through too late that the person has been tricking for a long time. Destructive exercise of power is also present when someone covertly relies on competition and fighting, but knows very well that he or she is dealing with a counterpart who still lives completely in the old value orientation (our altruists ► Chap. 1) and does not realize that the competitive orientation has taken over all areas of professional life. This person then relies on compromise-oriented communication rather than competition and struggle. Someone is also experienced as destructive, who in situations the largest profit for him- or herself, knowing well that the person opposite cannot or does not want to keep up there. In society as a whole, this kind of behaviour leads to a two-tier society with winners and an ever larger layer of those who cannot keep up or do not want to keep up.

Undeniably, power particularly attracts certain personality structures. As Alfred Adler (1927) believed, power is an excellent way to (over)compensate for feelings of inferiority. This need to turn a feeling of inferiority into superiority can be acted out in various ways, e.g. know-it-all attitude, striving for power, ambition. It is to be feared that no one will be deterred from doing so because of the risks that exist or are feared. Abuse of power can neither be prevented nor contained even by demonization of power. Demonization and tabooing even create additional free spaces for abuse and thus attract the "wrong" people.

This is another reason for facing up to the issue of power. On the one hand, we should understand this and try to harness it in a positive sense, and on the other hand, we should strive to put a stop to its abuse or excessive use through effective rules and control. In this way, the danger of corrupt systems forming can be countered.

In professional politics and psychotherapy, this "taming" of power takes place, for example, through regular elections, the strengthening of the position of patients and the creation of professional regulations. In the concrete psychotherapeutic situation, direct control from outside is not possible or even desirable. Indirect control results from the freedom to which both patients and psychotherapists are entitled, namely to terminate the treatment contract. In the meantime, Germany has a relatively good supply in the field of psychotherapy, so that patients do not have to fear that they will not get a new chance for therapy.

4.5.1 Forms of Destructive Exercise of Power in General

Destructive exercise of power in general and especially in psychotherapy is, in my opinion, given when destructive motives determine the actions.

These motives can be lived **consciously, openly** and **actively** in direct actions, e.g. by:

■ Assaults, Intimidation, Threats

Direct destructive power can be exercised through assaults, intimidation, threats, bullying, in order to experience oneself in the powerful position in any case. This usually involves a world view in which there must always be a superior and an inferior. Some then act according to the motto: Better to be guilty than powerless!

■ Bribery or Corruption

Destructive use of power can take the form of bribery or corruption to buy the silence or complicity of another. The more lucrative the "reward," the more seductive and corrosive it is to the other. There is an appropriate saying for this: send someone to the devil in such a way that they look forward to the journey.

- **Manipulation and Lies**

Manipulation and lying can be used to severely damage the reputation and integrity of another. If exculpatory witnesses are missing, even a real court conviction can be the result.

- **Revenge and Retribution**

Exercising power through revenge and retaliation can be the end result of a long chain. In the beginning, there may even be power struggles that have been won. But those who were defeated in these fights do not simply accept this, but open an open account: I'll get even with him/her. If the conflict was also unfair or conducted in a personally offending, devaluing and humiliating manner, then the superior is additionally resented. Own shares are often blanked out or reinterpreted as a reaction to the winner. The losers are waiting for a situation in which they can take revenge and retaliate without much risk.

- **Punishment as Revenge**

Furthermore, punishment can appear as revenge, e.g. for not providing support to a partner. The possibility for this arises the next time the partner is dependent on cooperation. Then he can be punished by refusing support or doing only what is necessary (rulebook slowdown) in order not to make himself vulnerable, or by covertly undercutting the project, spinning intrigues and possibly even watching with pleasure as the partner fights with growing desperation for his project and finally fails.

- **Ignorance as Revenge**

An often observed form of destructive exercise of power is ignorance as a form of revenge. With ignorance it is possible to let the other person run up from a safe cover or to set up barriers in the form of irrelevant doubts or additional tasks. If then the initiator of the project fails, it may have nothing to do with whether the project as such was worth it, but rather with the settlement of open accounts that arose in completely different contexts.

- **Denial**

Likewise, denial—especially the passive form—can be used as a not immediately perceptible but nevertheless sadistic means. Denial is a form often chosen by the perceived inferior to take revenge for actual or perceived wrongs. Even if it seems impossible in a situation to refuse support altogether (e.g., on the part of the patient because he or she wants to be treated, or on the part of the therapist because he or she feels obligated to provide care), one can decide how to provide that service. Intelligence and creativity can be used to mutual satisfaction or annoyance.

- **Boycott**

A boycott is perceived as particularly destructive if it is aimed at annoying and demotivating. Then the boycotter ostensibly propagates a good cooperation, but actually he only looks for what does not work and for whatever reasons it will never be able to work.

- **Sabotage**

Furthermore, as a further enhancement, use can be made of sabotage for the same motives. It is astonishing how much destructive energy in the form of intelligence and creativity is put into an action, the result of which is not only useless, but also realized in such a concealed way that not even an evil intention can be assumed. Then, when the other is beside himself with rage or despair, the saboteur takes great pleasure in the fact that his plan of revenge has succeeded.

- **Leave Open the Account**

It can go unnoticed for a long time that someone has left a score unpaid in order to continue to enjoy the feeling of secret superiority, because the other person is then trapped without knowing it. Someone with an unpaid bill has time on their hands. This revenge from "cold rage" is more dangerous and unpredictable than that from "hot rage." It can be assumed that many a top functionary, with whom many still have a score to settle, will then—unexpectedly for himself—fall when at some point the hour of reckoning arrives.

- **Insistence on Being Right**

A power struggle can develop for very different reasons, e.g. out of bossiness, in which the matter is then completely pushed into the background. Any disagreement, no matter how small, can develop into a power struggle if the argument turns into a fight for superiority. For example, if both are fully convinced that only their own opinion is right, there will be annoyance and anger on both sides and then a fierce conflict. And if then no one gives in, the power struggle is there.

- **Inferiority Power Struggle**

Basically, power struggles can develop not only from factual differences of opinion, but also from feelings of inferiority. If one partner does not take the other seriously, treats him condescendingly and exposes him ("You are a real cardboard nose"), then the other can put up with this (at the price of permanent belittlement) or he can fight. In the latter case, he enters a power struggle with an uncertain outcome. Sometimes it happens that no real, but only an imagined belittlement triggers someone to think that he has to re-establish his superiority or authority. Then it is "only" feelings and insinuations that trigger feelings of inferiority and the exaggerated reactions.

- **Power Struggle Out of Spontaneous Rejection**

Power struggles can also arise from spontaneous rejection, which can be so pronounced that one almost reflexively begins to fight the person concerned, whereupon he usually fires back. Seemingly without reason, fierce power struggles can arise. On closer inspection, it becomes clear that the antipathy arises because the other person embodies something that triggers hostile and/or fearful feelings at first glance. It is the inner resonance with the other that awakens certain thoughts, fantasies and feelings. And then rejection and devaluation can arise from spontaneous antipathy, e.g. someone can be perceived at first sight as threatening, as competition, envious, contemptuous.

Power Struggle in a Quest for Superiority

Sometimes a quest for superiority can turn into a power struggle between complete strangers. An example familiar to all is that of high-risk overtaking races on the motorway. People who don't know each other and didn't even know the other existed seconds ago get bogged down in a power struggle and forget the life-threatening quality of the situation. It's about dominance on both sides, and two different classes of motives can play a role: One is defensive in nature. Here, the actor is concerned with not allowing himself to be subjugated. It is often accompanied by a sense of self-defence. The other motive class is of an offensive nature. The other person should be made aware of one's own superiority, he should feel it. He is to be provoked, paraded and humiliated. He is to be punished for his misconduct (measured by one's own standards).

Power Struggle for Base Motives

It is particularly alarming when power struggles are conducted for base motives. Then the opponents are only concerned with establishing a pecking order. What prevents people from resolving conflicts through division and recognition? Adler (1927) suggests that all people, as social beings, strive to belong to a community and at the same time suffer from feelings of inferiority. Therefore, they do not feel that they belong to the community by nature, by birth, so to speak, but think that they have to earn this place first. The deeper the feeling of inferiority, the more vigorous the efforts. Adler speaks in this connection of overcompensation. According to him, we try to prove to ourselves and to others our own greatness and thus earn our place in the community. And the greater the self-doubt, the greater the need for proof at the expense of others. Arno Gruen (2016) sees the causes of these self-doubts and feelings of inferiority in a fundamental weakness of our culture's thinking, namely in the overemphasis on abstract and individualistic thinking: "Life as an expression of love, of empathic perceptions and compassion, is lost. In its place is a lurking fear of failure, of powerlessness, as the pursuit of security was based on meeting the expectations of parents and other authorities. And so people in our cultures are reduced to status and social position." (ibid., p. 95)

Territorial Thinking

Doubts and feelings of inferiority and, as a consequence, territorial thinking can be triggered even by trivial things. Usually it is not even about weighty factual questions or setting the course, when one tries "to assert one's own will even against opposition" (Weber 1922; ▶ Chap. 2), but about seemingly banal things like: "Who has the right of way?" or "Who said it first?" or "Who has not been asked?". With such questions there is no struggle for shaping power, but it is mostly only about the pecking order, about one's own importance. This is then again about behaviour that is mainly "ego-driven" and not "unbiased" motivated, which has a high price individually, in psychotherapy and in society as a whole.

Struggle for Personal Superiority and Validity

In extreme cases, the matter can then be misused as a legitimation and playing field for the struggle for personal superiority and validity. It is therefore important to distinguish between counterproductive power struggles and the constructive use of creative power. The use of shaping power is about the cause. In other words, one can examine a situation to see whether one is really concerned with achieving meaningful change and eliminating resistance in order to do so, or, for example, with being right. It can be appropriate to address blockers and objectors sternly, to impose conditions and—as a last resort—to exclude them. Power—properly motivated—will only be used when all other attempts to eliminate resistance have failed.

Almost all resistance, however, can be dissolved through empathy, firmness and communication. When it really comes down to it, iron determination and strong empathy are not a contradiction, but the two sides of the same coin.

So far, we have mainly dealt with the open, direct, usually also conscious forms of power struggle, because they are more conspicuous and spectacular. But the **indirect, passive, often unconscious destructive** means of power are not to be underestimated. Often they are even more destructive, more demoralizing and more effective than the overt ones.

■ Delay, Extenuation, Belittlement

Let's imagine a family with several teenage children. One parent A wants to enforce a different distribution of tasks, but all the children are against it, and the other parent B is rather neutral and indifferent to the project. After a few discussions, the parent A declares that he or she is no longer interested in these counterproductive discussions. At some point it would be over and the end of the debate. And then this parent orders the new distribution of tasks and does not go further into counter-arguments and objections. The eldest son, who had protested in particular, still has the daily garbage can emptying imposed on him. Let's assume that all other family members now realize that open resistance or protest is futile, but that does not mean that everyone has accepted the new distribution of tasks. We come to the point that everyone is writing a fat bill. Without having to agree, the family members now engage in an indirect, passive power struggle with parent A.

■ Compliments and Corruption

One child persists in simply keeping the previous, simpler tasks. When Parent A notices this, the child innocently tells A it's an exception: "I'm just helping my sister so there's no backlog." And that is also very good, helping each other, the child says.

■ Falsification, Manipulation

A child does something different than it should and explains that this is exactly what it should do.

■ Failure

The youngest does the new tasks so poorly that the parent would prefer to do them him- or herself immediately. The parent pulls himself together and explains the tasks repeatedly, but the result does not change.

▪ **Aggression Inhibition, Elicit Compassion, Use of Hydroelectric Power**

The youngest finally declares in tears, "I can't do it; I'm so clumsy; nothing I can do."

▪ **Excuses, Pretexts**

The other parent, who is not exactly thrilled about extra work either, leaves the new tasks for the time being "because of work overload in the company".

▪ **Paralysis**

When asked by parent A to please take care of it immediately, B says he or she is not clear about the task and asks if A can explain it to him or her again.

▪ **Filibustering**

When the task is finally completed after countless inquiries, A becomes aware that the task has been carried out to the letter and the result is largely unusable.

▪ **Ramp Up**

Parent A now receives messages from school that the middle child has not done his homework. The child says at school that he first had to do his chores at home and then did not have time to do his homework.

▪ **Refrigerate**

As the complaints from school and music school pile up and Parent B also begins to get restless, Parent A wonders who actually has the power in the household. A suspects that it is not him. Yet all the family members could have pulled out many more stops!

▪ **Refuse Empathy**

It is clear that the rest of our example family refuses to empathize with Parent A because they also felt left out and now (unconsciously) want revenge. This ironic, escalating satire can easily play out like this or similarly in reality, and it is then difficult for parents to find the beginning of the story.

Hannah Arendt named an incomparably more violent increase:

▪ **Banality of Evil**

Hannah Arendt (1963b) spoke of the banality of evil as a "surface phenomenon". It is characterized by the fact that someone has no motives except personal advancement, that obedience can justify everything, that there is an unwillingness to put oneself in the place of others, that empathy is downright denied. An important sign of this is the use of clichés (▶ Sect. 3.3.5): "In these last minutes it was as if Eichmann himself were drawing the conclusion of the long lesson in human wickedness that we had attended—the conclusion of the terrible 'banality of evil' before which words fail and thinking fails" (ibid., p. 371).

It is rare that people, including psychotherapists and patients, are aware, let alone declare, that they are exercising power in a destructive way. Yet, of course, it happens every day. "In therapeutic relationships, we are dealing with those that can mutate into perpetrator-victim relationships" (Piegler 2003, p. 107). In this context, power is always a relational phenomenon, because "power and powerlessness are two sides of a holistic phenomenon and are divided between the relational partners in the experience" (ibid., p. 108). In the following, conscious and unconscious forms of destructive exercise of power in psychotherapy are described—without claiming to be complete.

4.5.2 Forms of Destructive Exercise of Power By the Patient

How does destructive exercise of power on the part of the patient show itself concretely? Which personality weaknesses, which use of status and knowledge can produce destructive expressions of power? (The "tasks of the psychotherapist" attached to each example are explained in ► Chap. 5).

▪ **Personality**

For example, patients want to get the therapist to advocate for them and support them. This can be accompanied by (unconscious) fantasies of redemption. **Conscious or unconscious coercion** always thrives on the conviction that the other person will play along. Some patients exclude the possibility that they will be sent on and get into inner trouble when the therapist behaves differently than expected. They then build up moral pressure, for example. (Tasks of the psychotherapist: cognitive and emotional empathy and determination).

Conversely, patients develop a willingness to **"play along against their better judgment"** when the therapist suggests treatment and even when they themselves are not convinced. This may arise from fear of disappointing the therapist and may feel to patients as if they are saving themselves from a threat. Transference and regression can play a large role in these feelings and fears early on in a therapeutic process. At a borderline level, "playing along" can also consist of not showing one's feelings and views. This then reflects a diminished willingness to take responsibility and activity. In both cases, the ability or willingness to empathize with the other, the therapist's side, is lowered. (Tasks of the psychotherapist: Attention to contradictions and clarification).

As a therapist, one can observe that the more pressure patients are under, the more they look only at themselves, often (unconsciously) feeling the need to save themselves. They **cooperate out of fear** that the psychotherapist will harm them. They no longer even think about the interests and intentions of the other side. They then no longer notice that the supposedly powerful person does not want to harm them at all or is just as dependent on them and their cooperation as they are on him. (Tasks of the therapist: Stimulating alternative perspectives and selective self-opening).

Patients may consciously or unconsciously try to use their mentalizing ability in a manipulative way to control the psychotherapist's behaviour and feelings – so-called **misuse of mentalizing** (► Sect. 3.3.5). To do this, they use above-average cognitive empathy and anticipation skills, while emotional empathy appears to be below average or even non-existent. **Negating mentalization** also belongs in this spectrum. Patients deny, often politely, having anything to say about a question that stimulates self-reflection. They avoid giving concrete explanations to the psychotherapist. They usually justify actions with physical rather than mental-psychological conditions. (Tasks of the psychotherapist: Irritating questioning and attitude of not knowing).

Furthermore, patients can **hypo- as well as pseudo- and hypermentalise** (▶ Sect. 3.3.5), either by perceiving their own intentions and feelings or the motives and feelings of the psychotherapist too little or excessively. Excessive attributions can be, for example, the assumption of evil motives in the psychotherapist. (Tasks of the psychotherapist: Challenge and inquisitive stance)

It can be destructive when patients have such a strong ambivalent need for closeness that the moment contact is made or "threatened" by themselves or by the psychotherapist, the patient distances themselves with insults and humiliations, confusing to the point of discouraging the psychotherapist with these **attacks on linking** (Bion 1959). (Tasks of the psychotherapist: Understanding interaction in psychotherapy and interpreting).

The effect can be just as violent when patients express dissatisfaction and defiance about progress over a long period of time when the psychotherapist was actually expecting improvement. A **negative therapeutic reaction** is said to occur when a deterioration in the clinical state follows an important insight, signs of progress, or expressions of understanding and praise. Freud explained this phenomenon in terms of a strong unconscious sense of guilt that demands punishment through suffering. (Tasks of the psychotherapist: Patience and understanding of interaction in psychotherapy and interpreting).

It can bring both sides to despair if in the course of the cooperation (unconscious) feelings of powerlessness push from superficial or deeper layers in the patient, true to the motto "Never again powerlessness" go into the opposite and **show** the psychotherapist their **superiority and strength.** (Tasks of the psychotherapist: cognitive and emotional empathy and confidence building and determination).

It is particularly difficult in those rare cases when patients harbor unjustified distrust and suspicion not only of the psychotherapist, but also of all other people. They then basically assess their motives as malicious and attacking. In their **delusions, paranoia and fantasies of grandeur,** they feel they are under constant and unfair attack, attacks on their person, their dignity, their integrity, their good will. The relationship can easily derail, and conflicts can spread into the partnership, professional, economic and legal spheres. (Tasks of the psychotherapist: Working alliance and openness/transparency and containing).

▪ Status

Patients can, for example, because of their status, let themselves fall too much into the role of the one to be cared for and demand that the psychotherapist care for and support them. If developmental steps that would already be possible are then not taken or are prevented by strong regression, **malignant regression** is present. (Tasks of the psychotherapist: Understanding the interaction in psychotherapy and resource activation).

Similarly, patients or parents may insist on maintaining a disability status that could be overcome. This regressive refusal or prohibition may be an expression of addiction to **narcissistic gratifications or fixations on secondary illness gain.** (Tasks of the psychotherapist: Understanding the unconscious pathogenic belief and cognitive and emotional empathy and developmental support).

Normally, patient and therapist—much like a couple—seek their **form of togetherness** on a continuum between total fusion and rigid demarcation. In the case of total symbiosis (and the desire to enhance one's own status), the illusion of a shared self can form—with a strong demarcation from the outside world. There is then a danger of over-intimacy and a loss of one's own ego boundaries on both sides. With rigid demarcation, both strongly demarcate themselves from each other out of fear of loss of self (and loss of their own status) and a fear of closeness and intimacy. The demarcation to the outside is then often unclear, because the outside functions as a protection against too much closeness in the therapeutic relationship. (Tasks of the psychotherapist: self-object differentiation and clear boundaries).

Another form of destructive exercise of power described in the literature can be that patients' efforts to strongly idealize their psychotherapists initially turn into aggressive de-idealization later on. Some patients have the reputation of being **luminary killers** (Overbeck 1997; Kuiper 1980). Then the assumption is obvious that they want to enhance their own status by devaluing the other person. (Tasks of the psychotherapist: Clarifying, validating and simply intervening).

Patients may also attempt to enhance their own status or compensate for feelings of inferiority by bringing to bear **primitive defensive strategies,** e.g., mechanisms such as splitting, projective identification, denial, or strategies such as exploiting, lying, cheating. (Tasks of the psychotherapist: Analysis of the defense formation and emotional validation).

▪ Knowledge

Patients can use their knowledge for the purpose of influence. They try to create **massive pressure on the other person.** They explain eloquently, for example, that the psychotherapist must issue a statement, a certificate, an application for a cure, that they have no choice but to have this demand fulfilled by him, because otherwise they would not be granted a pension, a rehab, a cure, etc., i.e. they would have to suffer the most serious disadvantages. The fact that there are other people who could enforce such things even with the authorities cannot shake this certainty. The reference to it only triggers anger. (Tasks of the psychotherapist: Conflict readiness and clarity and empathy).

One can ask oneself, if one wants to understand the inner logic of this aggressively defended demand, what is the benefit of this behavior and what would be the alternatives. If these patients were to give up their conviction, they would have to risk conflict or admit their **lack of courage,** because those who risk conflict also risk defeat. These would then be suffered by the therapist. (Tasks of the psychotherapist: empathy and containing and reality reference).

In this way, patients can use their view of the world to justify their tendency to avoid conflict. This worldview shapes the way a person perceives and interprets a situation, what fears and catastrophic ideas he develops. He can then speak at length and with intellectual sophistication about the injustice of the world while at the same time **avoiding any conflict**. As a result, he may fall far short of his potential despite good education, good looks, and attractive offers. If psychotherapy fails to change this defensive formation, the price of fearful conflict avoidance is unsuccessful psychotherapy. (Tasks of the Psychotherapist: Confrontation and Interpretation)

The consequence is, among other things, that the patient is right in his prediction of being powerless and can then feast on his own **self-fulfilling prophecy.** Insisting on their powerlessness spares them the confrontation with others and thus the conflict as well as the risk of defeat. (Tasks of the psychotherapist: Insistence and refutation of the unconscious belief).

4.5.3 Forms of Destructive Exercise of Power By the Psychotherapist

What does destructive exercise of power on the part of the psychotherapist look like in concrete terms? Here, too, I structure the answer along the lines of weaknesses in personality, misuse of status and knowledge. (The "tasks of the psychotherapist" attached to each example are also explained in ► Chap. 5).

- **Personality**

For example, psychotherapists can subtly exercise destructive power out of a narcissistic problematic by appearing as seemingly **selfless helpers and heroes**, but in reality "helpless helpers" (Schmidbauer 1977). (Tasks of the psychotherapist: self-awareness and context analysis)

They can convey that they would be the **best helper in the world.** They live out their idealization desires and almost expect that every patient must fall in love with them. In such a constellation it can also come to sexual abuse. (Tasks of the psychotherapist: self-awareness/psychotherapy and abstinence)

Sometimes psychotherapists try to live out their unfulfilled **harmony and symbiosis desires** in their therapies. The more dissatisfied the therapist is with his private life, the more this happens. Symbiosis desires are often associated with the inability to regulate closeness and distance and to draw boundaries. (Tasks of the psychotherapist: self-awareness and development of the private life).

It is often difficult to recognize when psychotherapists unconsciously want to take revenge, e.g. due to a hidden hatred of a parent. These **desires for revenge** often camouflage themselves with fantasies of grandeur or rescue impulses. Patients who themselves have often been disappointed in their lives unconsciously perceive these narcissistic problems of the psychotherapist and burden therapists e.g. with feelings of hatred, which can considerably complicate the problem. (Tasks of the psychotherapist: self-experience/psychotherapy and context analysis).

The task of self-experience is to sensitize psychotherapists to act according to their **neurosis type** (Riemann 1961) ("► Neurosis Types").

Neurosis Types

The **schizoid therapist** expects healing through harmonious understanding. In conversation, he often shows an unyielding detective attitude, which makes it difficult for the patient to trust and which, on the other hand, maintains the unconsciously desired distance. Emerging transferences are immediately nipped in the bud out of fear of loss of identity. His excellent intuition bears the danger that the patient sees his boundaries violated and reacts paranoid.

The **depressive therapist** expects healing through the nurturing therapeutic relationship and thus at the same time participates in the patient's life. Together with a depressed patient, the danger of oral collusion arises (psychotherapist as inexhaustibly nurturing mother, patient as needy foster child). The therapist always fears separation from the object, i.e. fears that the patient will do without him. Therefore, he finds it difficult to allow the patient to engage in his own activities and to expand his competencies independently in and outside of the session. Confrontation is shied away from, therefore aggressive sides of the relationship have to be denied or projected.

The **compulsive therapist** expects healing by giving the patient the knowledge of what is "right" for him. He fights arbitrary and chaotic parts in the patient. Power plays a fundamental role in this, because the therapist is the one who thinks he knows what is "right" for the patient. There is a danger of anal collusion if the therapist tries to exercise as much power and control as possible over the patient who is dependent on him. As a result of the therapist thinking that his norms are the right ones, he has trouble thinking his way into the patient's system of norms and accepting them as equal.

The **hysterical therapist** is in danger of creating a phallic collusion. He wants to be admired and experiences this, for example, when he makes as many patients as possible fall in love with him. For the hysterical therapist, "working through" seems too tedious and boring. (Tasks of the psychotherapist: Knowing one's own type with strengths and weaknesses).

A **pathological fit** between patient and psychotherapist can have a particularly destructive effect. The pathological fit is fixed by transference and countertransference that cannot be understood and resolved. Bergmann-Mausfeld (2006, 2013) describes the phenomenon of pathological fit as an attachment to a pathogenic object. It represents the "underlying developmental conditions of an inadequately formed 'theory of mind' and the resulting psychodynamics with their intra- and interpsychic effects" (Bergmann-Mausfeld 2013, p. 459). The dependence on the pathogenic object is difficult to resolve because there is a fit in a pathological and tragic way that must be understood by the psychotherapist. (Tasks of the psychotherapist: structure building and establishment of good object representations and own supervision and if necessary self-experience).

As a further form of destructive exercise of power, psychotherapists—analogous to the experience of powerlessness of patients—can, if in the course of the collaboration an (unconscious) experience of powerlessness presses on them from superficial or deeper layers, true to the motto "Never again powerlessness" go into the opposite and **show** the patient unexpectedly and unsolicited their **superiority and strength.** (Tasks of the psychotherapist: Empathy and self-awareness and self-reflection).

Furthermore, psychotherapists may be at risk of creating narcissistic collusion (Willi 1975). In **narcissistic collusion**, the narcissist and co- or complementary narcissist meet for mutual satisfaction of their needs. One seeks and enjoys admiration and validation, the other experiences enhancement through demonstrated grandiosity. In this process, the narcissist and co-narcissist share the same psychological problems, namely high levels of vulnerability, longing for recognition and love, but each chooses a different way to compensate for their deficit. By identifying with the grandiose partner, the patient experiences enhancement via affiliation with that partner rather than for its own sake. Both roles are often gender-typed, i.e., the role of co-narcissist is taken by women who have **always** been **waiting for a "prince in shining armor"** to illuminate their lives through "his brilliance".

This constellation can increase if the psychotherapist has feelings of guilt due to his egoism and has **to repress them. Then aggression, craving for criticism** and severe humiliation of the co-narcissist **become apparent.** If he then sacrifices himself even more and becomes more submissive, the therapist's unconscious feelings of guilt intensify and prevent adequate self-criticism. Potentially, the more the other becomes a victim, the more he becomes a perpetrator—and vice versa. (Tasks of the psychotherapist: self-experience/psychotherapy and supervision and further education)

Another form of destructive exercise of power may be that psychotherapists try to compensate for feelings of inferiority by bringing to bear **primitive defensive strategies,** e.g. mechanisms such as splitting, projective identification, denial, or strategies such as taking advantage, lying, cheating. (Tasks of the psychotherapist: Analysis of one's own defense formation and context analysis).

In the worst case, psychotherapists—like patients—may also harbour unjustified mistrust and suspicion of other people. They then assess their motives as fundamentally malicious and attacking. In their **delusions, paranoia, and fantasies of grandeur,** they feel they are under constant and unfair attack, attacks on their person, their dignity, their integrity, their good will. The relationship can easily derail, and conflicts can extend into the partnership, professional, economic and legal spheres, as in a Folie à deux. (Tasks of the psychotherapist: self-experience/psychotherapy and working alliance and reality check/supervision).

▪ Status

For example, psychotherapists can exert **coercion** on patients in many different ways. They can try to enforce unrealistic expectations concerning the goal or the duration of the therapy by intrusively and manipulatively forcing the patient to open up to him/herself and thus undermine the patient's defences. (Tasks of the psychotherapist: reality reference and self-restraint).

There is an even greater danger for the patient when psychotherapists want to cultivate **dominance and fantasies of omnipotence.** It can develop from this that the patient's admiration and need for help causes an exaggerated sense of importance, irreplaceability, power and being needed. This entrenches the patient's suffering. (Tasks of the psychotherapist: self-experience and inclusion of multimodal working).

The profession of psychotherapist brings with it the danger that psychotherapists, by mentally dividing themselves into healthy and sick, become entangled in the assumption of a **healthy psychotherapist** and a sick patient. This assumption serves the therapist's defence against fear, but is counterproductive for the patient's developmental needs. (Tasks of the psychotherapist: questioning own norms and context analysis).

It is rare, but it does happen that psychotherapists take advantage of their status and **act as perpetrators.** According to a study by the Institute for Psychotraumatology Freiburg/Cologne, which takes into account the latest national and international research results, at least 300–600 sexual assaults must be expected annually in the Federal Republic of Germany. According to this minimum estimate, the statistical risk is less than 1% (German Institute for Psychotraumatology, 16.03.2016). However, in large American studies of 1000 psychiatrists and an equal number of psychologists, about 12% each admitted to sexual contact with their patients (cf. Piegler 2003). (Tasks of the psychotherapist: Psychotherapy and self-disclosure and, if necessary, acceptance of the withdrawal of the license to practice).

It happens that psychotherapists, taking advantage of their status, are in danger of **abuse of trust, ignorance, credulity, helplessness, economic hardship of patients**. Abuse of power in psychotherapy can develop insidiously. In the process, the patient's personal boundary and integrity are disregarded. The violation of boundaries can happen, for example, as manipulative indoctrination, when the therapist makes his own world view and understanding of reality absolute, by repeatedly making defamatory remarks, by excessive pessimism when the patient is thinking of dropping out of therapy, by black-billing fees, by disregarding the abstinence rule (not entering into private, professional or economic dependency relationships) and other types of emotional, verbal or structural violence. (Tasks of the psychotherapist: self-experience and context analysis and supervision).

It seems to be widespread that psychotherapists treat **relatives as "Transference related open season"** (Willi 1975, p. 253). Willi describes an often unrecognized abuse facet of the therapeutic two-way situation, namely collusion towards third parties, e.g. other therapeutic schools or relatives of the patient. In this process, the therapist shifts, for example, the negative reactions and aggressions that have arisen in his countertransference onto the relatives. "The relatives are (…) kept as Transference related open season. They may be shot down at will. It flatters many a therapist to feel superior, brave, strong and successful towards the relatives." Willi sees this triangular constellation as a late revenge for early Oedipal injuries. (Tasks of the psychotherapist: self-experience and context analysis and supervision).

▪ Knowledge

Psychotherapists may attempt to control patients through **mental** manipulation for the purpose of self-serving manipulation. Suggestions such as "You can believe me that … ", "I can assure you that … ", "There is absolutely no doubt in my mind that ... " show that the power of words is exploited to prevent the patient's thinking, to exaggerate facts or to generalize. An infamous tactic is to **deliberately** place subtle changes, distortions, generalizations. On the surface these inaccuracies look like minor mishaps, but they can drive the other person to despair or white heat, as when the patient has spoken of "problems" and the therapist refers to them as "challenges," when instead of "crises" they talk about "learning opportunities." (Tasks of the psychotherapist: self-experience/therapy and context analysis and strengthening of own integrity).

Psychotherapists must be careful not to use **psychologising** as a form of hyper- or pseudo-mentalising (► Sect. 3.3.5). In the "pretend" mode, thoughts and feelings can be discussed without the therapist being touched or processed internally or being able to induce processes of change. (Tasks of the psychotherapist: self-experience/therapy and integration of the pretend mode).

Already in the classical analytic literature it is pointed out that psychotherapists can misuse their knowledge by claiming an exaggerated **power of interpretation** or **interpretive sovereignty**, which can be understood as an abuse of mentalizing (the property of psychic states to be unclear [opaque] is not respected). Interpretive sovereignty means the concrete implementation of the "claim to the final say". With this claim to be able to interpret a subject correctly only oneself is connected the attempt to influence the opinion and feelings of the patient. (Tasks of the psychotherapist: Theoretical further education and confrontation with own narcissistic parts and structure building).

Freud already warns that practitioners succumb to a so-called healing mania, the **furor sanandi** (Freud 1915). "The psychoanalyst knows that he works with the most explosive forces and requires the same caution and conscientiousness as the chemist. (...) I am certainly not in favor of abandoning the harmless methods of treatment. They are sufficient for some cases, and after all, human society has no more need of the furor sanandi than of any other fanaticism. But it is to grossly underestimate the psychoneuroses, according to their origin and practical importance, to believe that these affections must be conquered by operations with harmless remedies." (ibid., p. 319f.). (Tasks of the psychotherapist: self-experience/therapy and self-reflection and supervision)

4.5.4 Forms of Destructive Exercise of Power By the System

As much as it is a progress that psychotherapy is covered by statutory and private health insurances and thus a fixed component of the general care of the population, one must not overlook or neglect the dark sides.

Patients must bear in mind that the assumption of costs by a health insurance company is always tied to the psychotherapist diagnosing a mental illness—currently according to ICD-10. For the conclusion of occupational disability, life and private health insurances, for example, there can be considerable risk surcharges or even an exclusion if psychotherapy has to be stated in the health check.

With a fixed schedule of probation, diagnostics and application procedure with report to the assessor and fixed quotas, a concrete psychotherapy is also an administrative process in which many people are involved as case workers. Sometimes, due to fear of precedents, lawsuits or too much responsibility, decisions are made that would have been different on an individual level.

In addition, there is continuous work at the political, professional and scientific levels to review and improve procedures, methods, quotas, qualifications, etc. In principle, these are sensible and productive efforts, but they can always mean hardship and unjustified restrictions for individual cases. For example, patients cannot assume that their health insurance will cover the number of sessions deemed necessary by the psychotherapist, as the guidelines provide for a clear limit.

Another problem can be the expert procedure/review, although it is currently the best procedure for protecting the therapist from recourse claims and for quality assurance. Psychotherapists have to invest a lot of time and energy in applying for psychotherapy. The report to the reviewer takes up most of this time. Even more burdensome for many is the risk of not being able to keep promises and then no longer being able to do justice to the patient if the expert does not approve.

The choice of psychotherapy procedure is also not up to the patient. But a so-called guideline-based treatment cannot be the means of choice for a particular patient. The Scientific Advisory Board on Psychotherapy (WBP), for example, is concerned with the development and updating of scientific criteria for the assessment of psychotherapeutic procedures or treatment methods and their application. As important as the scientific assessment of procedures is, any review of effectiveness is also influenced by professional political forces. For example, it was important to bring to the attention of the WBP that in the field of analytical psychotherapy "theoretically elaborated and empirically supported process and individual case studies (…) should be increasingly considered by the WBP" (Brandl et al. 2004, p. 14).

Even if training structures and the Psychotherapists Act have functioned stably over the last 16 years after decades of discussions and negotiations and did not seem to be shaken by anything, these structures have also been up for discussion on the political stage for some years now. Many associations, professional politicians and practitioners are critical of the plans to reform the training of psychotherapists and consider that these plans threaten the quality of psychotherapeutic care and training in Germany. These development tendencies illustrate in a particularly extreme way that nothing is secure and fixed, that every patient and every psychotherapist, lecturer, supervisor, institute director is also constantly exposed to and dependent on a potentially destructive play of forces. In this context, my impression is that in the field of psychotherapeutic professional politics, people often proceed with a verbally professed "political correctness", "strong aversion to conflict" and a lot of "diplomacy". Never would anyone at this level make the "mistake" of openly stating their opinion about the disadvantages of their own orientation or show their true motives. Everyone hides their true opinions behind a lot of verbal concession. When in doubt, it's all for more equity and for the good of patient care. Everyone assures one of support, but which fate the individual takes is ultimately uninteresting. This is what e.g. the countless lecturers and supervisors of the German training institutes had to realize and learn in the last years.

One advantage of the currently applicable training conditions for psychotherapists, which must be paid or earned postgradually by the prospective psychotherapist himself or herself, is that he or she has no obligation to repay or work off an investment by the state after completing training.

In everyday life it is clear to psychotherapists and patients that they cannot easily eliminate destructive tendencies resulting from certain decisions of the system, that they have to deal with them somehow. In terms of power politics, it then seems wise to "do things in a small way" when one is dependent on the go-along or goodwill of actors over whom one has no direct influence.

Whether one likes it or not, in such a case more than the individually available persistence and assertiveness and also more power politics are required to bring about fundamental changes.

Generally speaking, influencing overtly or covertly destructive aspects or areas of policy and professional politics is a longer journey that requires both a great deal of perseverance and considerable willingness to engage in conflict, and must be carefully tailored to the particularities of each organisation's and institution's culture, the further discussion of which would take us too far here.

The following chapter will focus on how to deal with destructive use of power in practice as a psychotherapist.

References

Adler A (1927) Menschenkenntnis. Menschenkenntnis. Fischer, Frankfurt a.M. 1966

Arendt H (1963a) Wahrheit und Politik. In: Wahrheit und Lüge in der Politik. Zwei Essays. Piper, München 1972

Arendt H (1963b) Eichmann in Jerusalem. Ein Bericht von der Banalität des Bösen. Piper, München, p 2011

Bergmann-Mausfeld G (2006) Pathologische Passung, Mentalisierung und negative therapeutische Reaktion. Forum Psychoanal 22:249–267

Bergmann-Mausfeld G (2013) Die Vertreibung aus der Hölle. Zur Bindungskraft früher pathogener Bindungserfahrungen. Forum Psychoanal 29:459–475

Bion WR (1959) Angriffe auf Verbindungen. In: Bott Spillius E (Hrsg) (1990) Melanie Klein heute, Bd. 1. Verlag Internationale Psychoanalyse, München, S. 110–139

Brandl Y, Bruns G, Gerlach A, Hau S, Janssen PL, Kächele H, Leichsenring F, Leuzinger-Bohleber M, Mertens W, Rudolf G, Schlösser AM, Springer A, Stuhr U, Windaus E (2004) Psychoanalytische Therapie. Eine Stellungnahme für die wissenschaftliche Öffentlichkeit und für den Wissenschaftlichen Beirat Psychotherapie. Forum Psychoanal 20:13–125

Freud S (1915) Bemerkungen über die Übertragungsliebe. GW X, S. 306–321

Greenson R (1967) The technique and practice of psychoanalysis, vol 1. International Universities Press, New York

Gruen A (2016) Wider die kalte Vernunft. Klett-Cotta, Stuttgart

Kraus B (2013) Erkennen und entscheiden. Beltz, Weinheim/Basel

Künkel F (1929) Die Arbeit am Charakter. Die neuere Psychotherapie in ihrer Anwendung auf Erziehung, Selbsterziehung und Seelenführung. Bahn, Schwerin

Künkel F (1935) Grundzüge der praktischen Seelenheilkunde. Hippokrates, Stuttgart

Kuiper PC (1980) Die seelischen Krankheiten des Menschen. Huber, Stuttgart

Moeller ML (1982) Sich selbst überleben. Kursbuch 70:71–99

Nietzsche F (1874) Unzeitgemäße Betrachtungen – Schopenhauer als Erzieher. Insel, Berlin, p 1981

Overbeck G (1997) Der Koryphäenkiller. Suhrkamp, Frankfurt a.M

Piegler T (2003) Macht, Ohnmacht und Machtmissbrauch in psychotherapeutischen Beziehungen. Psychotherapie Forum 3:106–112

Riemann F (1961) Grundformen der Angst. Ernst-Reinhardt-Verlag, München

Schmidbauer W (1977) Die hilflosen Helfer. Über die seelische Problematik der helfenden Berufe. Rowohlt, Reinbek bei Hamburg

Sterba R (1934) The fate of the ego in psychoanalytic therapy. Int J Psychoanalysis 15:117–112

Weber M (1922) Wirtschaft und Gesellschaft. Siebeck, Tübingen

Willi J (1975) Die Zweierbeziehung. Spannungsursachen, Störungsmuster, Klärungsprozesse, Lösungsmodelle. Reinbek bei Hamburg, Rowohlt

As a Psychotherapist, How Do I Deal with Destructive Use of Power?

Contents

M.-L. Althoff, *Mentalizing Power and Powerlessness*,
https://doi.org/10.1007/978-3-662-66119-2_5

At the beginning of this chapter, the question is answered as to what strategies and interventions one has at one's disposal as a psychotherapist in order to be able to get out of one's own destructive power behaviour or to prevent the patient from exercising destructive power or to escape a mutually destructive exercise of power. The dynamics of destructive, perverse power scenarios are then examined, which are themselves understood as a heightened form of destructive power exercise and are characterized by destructive power being exercised more permanently, frequently, repeatedly to the point of sadism, callousness, cruelty, or ruthlessness. How to understand and cope with such power scenarios is discussed. Only after an exit from the destructive or perverse power scenario can deeper mentalizing steps be initiated. The then potentially helpful intervention possibilities of MBT are presented.

If one looks at everyday (therapeutic) life, one can observe that the two aspects of constructive and destructive exercise of power cannot be so strictly separated. Moreover, there are interactions between the constructive and destructive exercise of power. Motives are always multiform and multi-layered. Objective and ego motives often overlap in everyday life. For example, the pursuit of objectively justified goals can be mixed with questionable elements such as devaluation, punishment or dominance. This mixture, or one could say: contamination, is then detrimental to the cause.

No one can absolve himself of occasionally losing patience after several friendly but futile efforts to convince and motivate. It becomes even more problematic, however, when an ego-like, self-satisfied component is additionally mixed into the factual use of power and also the loss of patience, e.g.: "I'll show that deadbeat to stick it to me!".

As understandable and comprehensibly relieving as such a derailment can be in moments of pressure, it is not helpful. Because when the affected person hears or is told about this reaction, he will inevitably react to the devaluation, insult and humiliation contained in the remark. He understandably feels unfairly treated, feels hurt and belittled, and usually develops great anger and fantasies of revenge. If the affected person sees himself on the same or a higher level, he may choose the open power struggle. However, if he sees himself in the hierarchically lower position, he will not dare an open confrontation as a rule. His compensation then goes into indirect, passive forms of power struggle, such as the strategies of rulebook slowdown, passive refusal and covert sabotage mentioned in ▶ Chap. 4. The matter has then become secondary.

One can say that the following rule of thumb applies: The stronger and more unjust the personal humiliation triggered by the ego-based use of power is felt, the more compensatory energy is mobilized and the more violent is the subsequent, mostly passive, refusal. Conversely, the more appropriate the use of power, the more likely it is to be accepted by those affected. There is not always great enthusiasm, but at least there is no need for revenge. In this respect, it is worth disciplining oneself when using power, not only for moral and ethical reasons, but also in the interest of the cause, and to consciously refrain from taking out one's own frustrations or bad moods on others.

5.1 What Strategies and Interventions Do I Have at My Disposal as a Psychotherapist?

As part of the answer to the question of what strategies and interventions I have at my disposal as a psychotherapist to find a way out of destructive use of power, I first name four strategies that are useful and effective in psychotherapy, but also in human coexistence in general.

5.1.1 Constructive Communication

Once someone has a desire for revenge, it is practically hopeless to prevent or avoid all situations that enable that person to exercise overt or covert revenge. The only way to counteract the desire for revenge on the part of others is to give as little cause for it as possible. This does not mean always doing everything others want, or only being pleasant to others, or not opposing opposition from others, but it does mean creating as little unpaid bills as possible in one's own long-term interest. This is not about constant subordination, conformity and accommodation, and avoiding conflict, but about dealing and communicating in a way that is based on respect and mutual appreciation. As mentioned earlier, anger and rage and subsequent impulses for revenge usually arise not from what is done or represented, but from **how** it is done. Even if someone has to give in to a conflict, there will not automatically be a need for revenge-even if there is fear and disappointment-if the actions of the relationship partner seem transparent and fair. The need for revenge arises from the experience of arbitrariness, unpredictability, disregard, disrespect, belittlement. In order to shape change or decision-making processes, it is not enough to proceed logically and appropriately, but to communicate this logic clearly and appreciatively, in direct communication with those affected and over the entire period of time. Constructive communication is therefore a goal that accompanies the entire process. This requires, among other things, the courage to lead the conversation.

5.1.2 Conducting Interviews

If egoistic motives instead of appropriate considerations determine the actions, these motives must be uncovered in the conversation, because only in this way can a cooperation be continued without further emotional or material damage occurring or the destructive behavior drawing circles and affecting other people, e.g. in a family therapy. However, this is undoubtedly a demanding undertaking. If you get straight to the point by saying, for example, "Could it be that what you are doing is revenge for offenses that I have caused you by my behavior?", the other person will probably feel caught out, threatened, and insecure. Nevertheless, this is precisely the point, namely to address the suspicion that someone wants to take revenge or—to put it more weakly—"get even" or "give something back" in a calm and accepting conversational atmosphere and at a time that seems appropriate.

You have to be able to bear the fact that the other person may at first act indignant, as if the question were completely impertinent and out of line. If you then remain calm and express that you are not addressing the other person's behaviour with an intention of retaliation, openly addressing the other person's possible motive for revenge can have a relieving effect. It may even be possible to discuss what originally struck or offended him about the conversation initiator's behavior. Perhaps the person concerned will not openly admit what his motives were or are until the end of the conversation, but after the conversation it is also clear to him that he can no longer continue as before. In psychotherapy, such conversations happen within the therapeutic setting. In other settings, it may be useful and necessary to involve a mediator. If such destructive motives and subsequent actions can neither be discussed nor changed, it may be that the problem can only be solved by separation.

5.1.3 Recognition and Conscious Handling of Social Goals

What constructive social goals do people normally pursue, and what must happen for these to fade into the background or no longer come into play? Dreikurs (2009), a student of Adler, refers to his idea of the original "being ordered" to the community. He differentiates four basic social needs:

- the need to belong and feel loved,
- the need to experience oneself as capable, powerful and influential and to be important to others,
- the need to be respected and treated fairly,
- the need to feel safe, to be able to ask for help and to have the courage to take risks.

According to Dreikurs, those who feel accepted and belonging in these four areas of need behave constructively and actively contribute to the common cause. If these basic social needs are not met, Dreikurs concludes from his studies of children and adolescents, then they try by all means to achieve these goals after all and refer to the so-called disruptive proximal goals.

This begins with focusing attention on oneself and setting as a goal to improve one's position. Then comes the tendency to criticize and belittle others and oneself. The insecurity and lowered self-esteem may lead the person to the idea of forcing attention in less constructive ways. In such a situation, to insist that children need to be more obedient usually has the opposite effect, because it is not the child's lack of conformity that is the problem, but the lack of opportunity for creativity brought about by the adult's actions, and the increased pressure to conform triggers the (supposedly character-based) disobedience.

Dreikurs (2009) has found four recurring patterns that children and adults display: the disruptive or mistaken proximal goals. Many children come to therapy or are sent to treatment by parents, educators, and/or teachers because of these patterns. One or more patterns are evident in those concerned.

Disturbing or Erroneous Proximate Goals (According to Dreikurs)

- The person concerned (unconsciously) wants to force attention, recognition and service, e.g. by excessive self-display, conspicuous behaviour, by whining and complaining and by hypersensitivity.
- They (unconsciously) want to establish power and superiority, e.g. through know-it-all attitude, lying, belittling and devaluing others, stubbornness, constant opposition and rebellion, demonstration of supposed superiority or (passively) through petty insistence on rules and problematizing suggestions.
- They (unconsciously) seek revenge and retribution, e.g. punishing those around them for actual or perceived wrongs, thwarting others' plans, lustfully rejecting others' suggestions, scheming, sabotaging, and spreading suspicion, or (passively) by mistrusting, running down others, and not sharing information.
- They are permanently in (unconscious) denial, i.e. do nothing or only what is necessary, refuse everything new, feign inability and failure, withdraw, radiate resignation and drag others down with them.

Unfortunately, the overall reaction to these patterns in others is negative. The pattern Attention triggers anger and aversion. One step harsher are the reactions to the pattern Striving for Superiority. It triggers anger and rage and often causes others to enter into a power struggle. One step harder still are the reactions to vendettas. Even more anger and also indignation arise, especially when the other person has to put up with them and they have been engineered in such a way that you not only have to impotently put up with them, but also cannot fight them off. Fatally, this creates a new open account and thus the danger of an escalation of revenge. Finally, the fourth pattern, denial and failure, no longer triggers strong feelings. After perhaps initial anger and despair, the other person will feel only resignation and discouragement. All in all, the four types of provocation may achieve what the person wants in the short term—attention, superiority, revenge or denial—but they do not achieve a positive effect on acceptance and belonging.

The explanations for such behaviours open up perspectives for solutions, because the deeper causes of the provocative behaviour can then be recognised and worked through with the person concerned (in psychotherapy). In this respect, it is first necessary to realize that one should refrain from reacting spontaneously or intuitively to these disturbing social goals. One would then only run the risk of getting into anger and rage up to indignation and ultimately even getting involved in a power struggle. In doing so, one would be doing exactly what the unconscious intention of the person concerned is, namely to get involved in an interpersonal entanglement through the (negative) attention up to a power struggle and thoughts of revenge and a refusal. By doing so, one does not solve anything, but only creates an additional problem when one then gets involved in a destructive argument, for example.

The first two disruptive proximal goals, seeking attention and seeking superiority, can often be countered by simply giving the person encouragement and strengthening their sense of belonging. When it comes to revenge or denial, the suspected connections must be called by name. It will then become clear what can still be clarified in normal everyday life and when psychotherapy is necessary. With all hidden and unconscious revenge and refusal actions that cannot be addressed, it will come down to psychotherapy or a change of situation, e.g. dismissal, change of class.

5.1.4 Constructive Debate Instead of Power Struggles

Power struggles are one of the most difficult problems of interpersonal, family, school, company and psychotherapeutic everyday life, because they cause immense economic and human damage. For example, if someone in a conversation feels they have been treated inappropriately, suddenly neither the topic at hand nor how important the outcome of the conversation might be to all involved is of any interest. In this sense, disruptions always take precedence, whether or not they are addressed immediately and consciously. However, the reaction to actual or perceived disruptions easily builds up into a power struggle, because these disruptions usually spread an aggressive or devaluing mood. When it comes to the retaliation, the power struggle is there.

Power struggles are indeed legitimate between rival persons, if it is a matter of competition in which everyone has a chance. Nevertheless, it must be remembered that the relationship between the opponents is strained after one power struggle, and even more so after several. People then become more cautious, more sensitive to sidetones, they no longer inform each other, they avoid each other, they avoid issues. And the quality of the relationship, the trust and the results go down. At worst, you block and sabotage each other not overtly, but covertly. And then it's only a matter of time before even neutral third parties are functionalized and spun into intrigue. In my opinion, the disadvantages of power struggles to enforce interests are obvious. Moreover, changes generate so much anxiety and resistance even without a threatening gesture that there is no need to increase it by unnecessary power struggles. The more people feel threatened, the more they try to get out of harm's way or to get rid of the threateners.

> It makes more sense and saves resources to ensure a climate in which fears, concerns and objections can be openly discussed. What can be discussed openly does not have to be fought out via (covert) power struggles.

In addition, the person in charge can usually trust that if he or she has done everything possible to fully convince colleagues or (family) members or employees of the need for change and to prepare them, then ultimately the use of power against blockers and saboteurs will also find understanding and acceptance.

No one is immune to exercising power or engaging in power struggles in a destructive way from time to time. This fact is probably a phenomenon of our civilization, for there seems to have been less frequent and less destructive warfare in early cultures than in civilized societies (Freud 1932; Fromm 1976; Gruen 2016). We today cannot always perceive life as an expression of love, of empathic perceptions and compassion.

> In its place is a lurking fear of failure, of powerlessness, as the pursuit of security was based on meeting the expectations of parents and other authorities. And so people in our cultures are reduced to status and social position. (Gruen 2016, p. 95)

However, we can only speak of a destructive process in the sense of permanent destruction if it is enduring, frequent and constantly repeated. I will discuss this category of destructive perverse exercise of power and ways of getting out of it in ► Sect. 5.2. First of all, we will deal with strategies for coping with the "normal" destructive exercise of power, which every normal neurotic person also knows to a greater or lesser extent: being fatally offended, fits of rage and anger, insulting others, throwing objects, short-term perverse thoughts and actions of revenge, e.g. in separation situations. It is characteristic that after such situations the person asks himself how it could have come so far, develops feelings of guilt and apologizes if necessary.

5.1.5 Strategies for Destructive Use of Power by the Psychotherapist

Of course, psychotherapists have a special responsibility towards their patients and are obliged to immediately put an end to any form of destructive exercise of power that they recognise in themselves and, if necessary, to ask a trusted person for advice and help. With such a high standard, it is not easy to consciously address one's own destructiveness. Presumably, those who absolve themselves of *any* destructive exercise of power will taboo or deny their own destructive exercise of power and then tend to resort to the indirect, passive and unconscious destructive means of power (► Sect. 4.1). In this respect, the initial step out of one's own destructive exercise of power is to acknowledge the fact that we all act destructively from time to time. If you can then turn to the subject consciously, it makes sense to ask yourself what weaknesses in your own personality might lead to destructive behaviour or where you might fear an abuse of your own status and knowledge (► Sect. 4.3).

► Example

Let us assume that psychotherapist Bislang-Sorglos wonders why patients in general are so reluctant to be questioned, at least that is his own experience. Yet he knows that he can ask precise and objective questions and is also careful and good at logical reasoning. He thinks that his strength is that patients can expect coherent insights and analyses from him.

He now wants to investigate where he is probably in danger of exercising power destructively because of his personality. He knows from various feedback and his own assessment that he has some schizoid traits. He often seeks empathic harmonious understanding. He feels particularly on "the same wavelength" with Patient Vorsicht-Grenze, a 39-year-old lawyer. He feels that he is similar to him.

Suddenly he remembers a situation from last week's session. The patient was pleased with the empathic harmonious understanding of the psychotherapist and said with a smile, "It should always be like this. You understand me because we are so alike." The psychotherapist recalls feeling a little uncomfortable for a brief moment, thinking, "We're not that similar." (In retrospect, in supervision, he thinks he may have feared losing his own identity). His conscious thought was, "Now I want to know exactly what the patient means by that." And inquired down to the last detail and probed and probed. The patient's smile disappeared, he asked with a worried, somehow suspicious look: "I only meant that. What are you getting at now?" and gave only monosyllabic answers. Bislang-Sorglos noticed this, but somehow felt more comfortable again, even though he didn't know what had happened. After a little pause, the patient said, "My mother was always so intrusive." And told a story the psychotherapist already knew. Mr. Bislang-Sorglos became uncomfortable again, and said, "I think I asked so many questions, I felt like your mother." (In supervision, he realizes that he tends to immediately nip emerging transferences in the bud in an interpretive way out of concern for loss of identity). The patient Vorsicht-Grenze replied, "Yes, it could be, but that's all I know about it. We don't need to go through this any further either." (The psychotherapist gets an inkling in supervision that his good intuition, with which he immediately grasps transferences, contains the danger of boundary violation towards the patient).

Psychotherapist Bislang-Sorglos senses, as he recalls this sequence of the session, that the session somehow ended with a latent irritability on the part of the patient. He considers that he himself may have triggered this irritability. He reflects on his countertransference (feeling similar to the patient, several times feeling uncomfortable in the session) and his actions (intrusive questioning and quick interpretation) but then gets stuck, thinking, "Somehow I can't get it together." He decides supervision is probably a good idea. In supervision, Supervisor Hat-Ideen and Mr. Bislang-Sorglos hypothesize about how the patient processed his interventions. On the drive home, Mr. Bislang-Sorglos is preoccupied with his feelings of anger at himself and his own shame, and he ponders how he should probably approach Mr. Vorsicht-Grenze in the next session. (How Mr. Bislang-Sorglos then intervenes concretely in the psychotherapy is presented in ► Sect. 6.2). ◄

- **Self-help Strategies in Case of Own Destructive Exercise of Power**

- Recognition of the possibility of one's own destructive exercise of power, e.g. reality check
- Observation of countertransference, e.g. feelings of fusion or strong anxiety, working alliance, questioning own norms
- Self-reflection, e.g.: When was what and in which situation? What have I done?
- Help, e.g. abstinence, self-restraint, strengthening one's own integrity, confrontation with one's own narcissistic parts, structure building, self-experience, therapy (development of good object representations), supervision
- Measures, e.g. multimodal working, development of private life, self-indictment, withdrawal of licence to practise medicine/psychotherappy
- Further education, e.g. literature, seminars with self-experience components (recognising neurosis type and defence formation)
- Context analysis (► Sect. 6.1), e.g.: How did the patient process my action?
- Intervention in psychotherapy, e.g. finding words towards the patient
- Postprocessing, e.g.

  - Acknowledging what it was, e.g. dominance, manipulation, injury, slight.
  - Acknowledge that this has had an impact, e.g. feeling inferior, grief.
  - Development of cognitive and emotional empathy for oneself
  - Admitting one's own motives, e.g. feeling superior, need for distance
  - Admitting anger at oneself, shame and, if necessary, grief.
  - Forgive oneself and find a way to deal with feelings of guilt
  - Acknowledging one's own uncertainty about how to deal with the patient
  - Enduring one's own neediness, e.g. after forgiveness by patients
- Finding back into one's own strength (► Chap. 7), e.g. stabilising self-esteem

5.1.6 Strategies in Case of Destructive Use of Power by the Patient

Patients can act as they wish or as it occurs to them within the agreed setting. Nevertheless, situations can arise in which psychotherapists have the impression that "it can't go on like this", that the treatment is at an impasse or quandary. It is then often not easy to recognise the (unconscious) mechanisms of influence by the patient and then to react to them in an appropriate way.

► Example

It is about the patient Versorg-Mich, who was 19 years old at the time and had graduated from high school the previous year. She came to therapy because she often felt incompetent, insecure and weak. She had the impression of not being able to understand others, not being able to see through relationships and not being understood herself. The psychotherapist Verständnis-Gern noticed at first that she gave this patient comparatively much support and encouragement. In retrospect, it also became clear to her that the patient had always reacted with joy, great gratitude and a mild admiration. She took note of hints about development possibilities, perspectives and requirements, but did not elaborate on them. Mrs. Verständnis-Gern had more and more the feeling of being stuck in a dead end.

In one session, she realized how annoyed she had become with her role as the understanding, caring therapist. At the same time, she also realized that with this patient she usually talked more than usual, and wondered why.

She suddenly remembered a passage from an essay by Sandler (1976) in which he reported on a treatment in which he had talked more than he usually did. He wrote that after some time of reflection he had noticed that the patient usually raised his voice a little at the end of his remarks, as if he were asking a question, although he was not asking any questions. With this little change—according to Sandler—the patient succeeded, without consciously intending it, in getting him to talk comparatively much.

The psychotherapist considered it possible that her patient was unconsciously practicing the same thing. By getting the therapist to talk a lot and offer a lot of understanding by her standards, she lost the fear that her counterpart, i.e. the psychotherapist, would stop caring for her. However, if she continued to be available to the patient in this way, she would remain satisfied but "small, insecure, and incompetent." If, however, she were to refuse, and then possibly at once, the patient would feel all the more so, and would also feel ashamed and offended.

The psychotherapist found the courage to address the situation as simply as possible, without immediately having a competent and omniscient solution at hand, while keeping the working alliance in mind. (How the psychotherapist intervened in concrete terms is described in ▶ Sect. 6.3). ◀

▪ Strategies for Destructive Use of Power by the Patient

Character Traits:

- Determination
- Patience
- Conflict Readiness
- Reality reference
- Perseverance
- Love of Truth
- Courage and willingness to take risks

Therapeutic stance:

- Attention to contradictions
- Empathy
- not-knowing stance
- Questioning attitude
- Confidence Building
- Working Alliance
- Openness/Transparency
- Clear boundaries
- Clarity

Interventions:

- Empathic validation
- Clarification
- Confrontation
- Interpretation
- Stimulate alternative perspectives
- Selective self-opening
- Irritating questioning (in the sense of disturbing the system)
- Challenge
- Understanding interaction in psychotherapy (context analysis; ▶ Sect. 6.1)
- Holding
- Containing
- Resource Activation
- Understanding the unconscious pathogenic belief
- Refuting the unconscious pathogenic belief
- Development support

- Self-object differentiation
- Simply, unpretentiously intervene
- Emotional validation
- Defense Analysis
- Stimulate mentalization
- indicate limits

Measures:
- Setting limits
- Supervision
- Separation

5.1.7 Strategies in the Event of Destructive Use of Power on Both Sides

The destructive exercise of power on both sides has been staged in many movies. I would like to mention a very well-known comedy ("What about Bob?") as an example.

What About Bob? (1991): The Story of a Narcissistic Collusion
Dr. Leo Marvin believes he has reached the pinnacle of success. His new book, Baby Steps, is a bestseller, and a television crew wants to come to his vacation home for a live interview. Just before he leaves, a new patient, Bob Wiley, shows up at his practice. Leo wants to get rid of him quickly, just presses his new book into his hand and leaves for vacation (**destructive exercise of power on Leo's side**: attempt to cold Bob; narcissistic collusion; pseudo-mentalizing and abuse of mentalizing; splitting healthy psychotherapist and sick patient).

But Bob believes he has found the savior in Dr. Marvin and travels after him on vacation. Dr. Marvin tries to get rid of Bob, but Bob just won't let himself be shaken off (**destructive exercise of power** on **Bob's part**: exercise of coercion; narcissistic collusion; primitive defense mechanisms).

Leo's family takes more and more liking to Bob and his originality. Bob also intervenes in the live interview. Leo is so unnerved that he sends Bob to the psychiatric ward. However, everyone there is also taken with Bob. Completely desperate, Leo has to pick him up again. The story takes its course when Bob meets Leo's sister Lily and finally wants to marry her. Leo tries in vain to kill Bob, and eventually ends up catatonic in a mental institution. When his family comes to pick him up for Bob and Lily's wedding reception, he is able to break free.

In everyday therapeutic life, of course, the destructive exercises of power on both sides are usually much more subtle and unspectacular than in Bob's case, and one has to direct one's attention quite consciously to these often apparently quite incidental phenomena.

▶ **Example**

The father of one patient, Mr. Nie-Schuld, had reported that he was always having heated arguments with superiors and colleagues at work, and more recently with his son's teachers, although he found that these fights did not originate with him, for he always tried to meet the expectations placed on him by the persons concerned. He came to the session with clear signs of stress, excused his wife, and added, "But I'll tell her everything." He then almost ran into the treatment room, sat down quickly, and immediately looked expectantly at the psychotherapist, Ms. Genau-Genommen. The latter felt almost compelled by his look to follow and sit down particularly quickly, expecting him to start now, but to her astonishment there was at least half a minute's silence. The psychotherapist then said something first: "What would you like to talk about today? You know I always wait to see what you've brought." The father grinned, "Well, you've started now." Psychotherapist: "But only because you looked so long."

If, at the beginning of a conversation, the gaze of one person A falls on another person B, and A notices that B was already looking at her when she turned her gaze to B, then there is a social agreement that the person A who turned her gaze takes the speaker role and the other person B, who had already turned her gaze, takes the listener role. Thus, by turning one's gaze to another, one can assign the role of speaker and place oneself in the position of listener.

The psychotherapist now considered that the father had done exactly that, whether consciously or unconsciously, and could now actually have expected her to say something. But she had remained silent, or rather had initially refused to speak, because she thought that he should begin in accordance with the agreed ground rule. And when she spoke, in her opinion, she was at the same time violating the ground rule itself by referring to it. It was a silent struggle over who should speak first or who could force the other to speak. She wanted to get out of this power struggle.

The psychotherapist thinks about the initial situation: On the one hand, the situation was determined by social agreements, and there they are both on the same level. On the other hand, they had agreed on the ground rule that determines an assignment to the role of the patient (father) and to the role of the psychotherapist, possibly experienced by both as an assignment of "below" and "above", i.e. in the sense of dominance and submission. Which law is more valid, the bourgeois one, to which both have to subordinate themselves in the same way, or the therapeutic one, which came about at the suggestion of the therapist? The psychotherapist recognizes her own striving for dominance as well as the father's challenge. She senses determination. She thinks that she should approach the father with a questioning attitude and could stimulate in him (and in herself) an alternative view, i.e. to say, for example, that in an agreement it is actually irrelevant who originally proposed it. She might also be able to interpret how the power entanglement happened in the therapeutic interaction, possibly similar to other situations in everyday life. (How the psychotherapist intervened in concrete terms is described in ▶ Sect. 6.3). ◀

▪ Strategies for Destructive Use of Power on Both Sides

Here, the self-help strategies for one's own destructive use of power and the strategies for the patient's destructive use of power must be applied simultaneously. Being aware of this reduces the danger of looking only one-sidedly at the patient or oneself.

To avoid any misunderstanding: This book does not argue that destructive use of power should always be nipped in the bud and that a concrete exit should be found as soon as possible if it has already happened. Rather, psychotherapeutic situations in which destructive exercise of power becomes apparent can be used to reflect on further goals, unfavourable relationship constellations in the past and present, circumstances that cause illness and one's own involvement in them, on wishes and dreams. Only when destructive exercise of power has reached the stage that permanent subjective suffering of the patient or psychotherapist or the reference system of both has set in or is threatening, then concrete thought should be given to an early or immediate exit from this scenario. This is the case, for example, when a highly aggressive, permanent destructive exercise of power takes place within the framework of a destructive perverted power scenario. The destructive perverse exercise of power knows—as mentioned—also every normal-neurotic person more or less. However, it occurs only rarely and in extreme situations, and afterwards it immediately triggers the question of the person himself, how it could have come so far, triggers feelings of guilt and, if necessary, a need to apologize. In contrast, the person who permanently exercises destructive, perverted power never questions himself, never apologizes, and never seeks responsibility from himself. To shed light on this area and to speak of aggressor and victim does not mean that in such situations it is not at the same time considered important to think psychodynamically, to struggle for a neutral stance, and to pay attention to transference and countertransference. But it is, if necessary, just as important in the first instance,

- to get oneself to safety,
- to keep up one's own strength,
- to be unkind,
- Contacting third parties,
- to recognize destructive mechanisms in oneself and others,
- To be able to confront someone and not show emotional empathy,
- clearly: Empathy can't beat emotional coldness (Anyone who thinks that ends up in powerlessness and is thus part of the scenario again),
- clearly: Mentalizing can't beat non-mentalizing (Anyone who thinks that ends up in powerlessness and is thus part of the scenario again),
- in extreme cases, the involvement of the judiciary and lawyers can not be ruled out.

5.2 Ways Out of Destructive, Perverse Power Scenarios

"It is difficult to resist a violence that is neither tangible nor provable, and yet that hurts," writes Hirigoyen (2002) in the blurb of her book, "Die Masken der Niedertracht". She names in clear words the phenomena and prevalence of mental violence in everyday life.

> One human being can actually destroy another through continued mental torment, which can justifiably be called "psychic murder". We have all witnessed such attacks at various levels, between a couple, within families, in workplaces, or even in political and social life. Yet our society proves blind to this form of indirect violence. Under the pretext of tolerance, people become lenient. (ibid., p. 9)

Certainly, as mentioned, none of us can absolve ourselves of having acted "perversely" from time to time in an angry and hostile manner, and also possibly having felt schadenfreude or sadistic pleasure in the process. However, the process becomes destructive only through frequency and repetition (ibid., p. 11). In the following, I will outline the phenomena of perverse mental exercise of power as well as name an effective way of dealing with it.

Aggressions are subtle, often take place in private, there are hidden messages, there are no explanations for incomprehensible, unpredictable behavior, you can find humiliation, contempt, fear, distortion of reality, sadistic triumph, negation of values, norms and tradition. If these relationship characteristics determine life not only temporarily and in crises, but for a long time and permanently, one can speak of destructive-perverse relationship formation. Then not love but hatred, possibly also hatred of love (Hurni and Stoll 1999) is the basis of the relationship, at least on the part of the aggressor. Then it is the task of the attacked to recognize that he or she can do nothing to change this, i.e., he or she must recognize his or her powerlessness. To make matters worse, the attitude of justification and defense drives the victim to engage in behaviors that irritate or are experienced by those around him or her as odd because the controlling influence is not visible to outsiders. "The environment does not understand and is seduced into a negative opinion of the victim" (Hirigoyen 2002, p. 120). Often the powerlessness and hopelessness goes so far that "only the law (daaaaa000p…) can limit the scope of violence" (ibid., p. 49). In court disputes and divorce proceedings, however, it is often difficult even for judges to recognise who is manipulating whom, and they themselves then worry about becoming victims of manipulation.

The victim's ability to respond is blocked (ibid., p. 80ff), among other things by.

- Refusal to communicate,
- Belittling and insulting,
- Treat as a thing-object,
- Exploiting strength and skills,
- Discredit in the presence of others,
- Isolate,
- Hazing,
- Causing the other person to make mistakes,
- Playing up mistakes,
- sexual harassment and assault,
- physical violence.

Power in the hands of unscrupulous people is so terrible because they make use of their weapons in a figurative and real sense.

Perverse Machinations of the Attackers (Examples)

- Use of charm and attractiveness
- Use of authority
- Create weakness by paralyzing the victim
- produce fear

- Beckon with rewards (family) or promotion (company)
- sow self-doubt
- Exploit confusion and depression
- Making overt or covert threats
- Communication as prevention of exchange
- Fear inducing language and timbre
- Lies, mockery, contempt
- Imposing, not keeping distance
- In the final stage: open hatred, violence, reversal of good and evil, delusion

The Consequences for the Attacked Person

- Initially: refraining from conflict management
- Negative sides are seen, but other sides are idealised instead
- disruption of faculties
- Losing your own self-esteem
- One's own doubt ("Am I really capable of nothing?")
- Environment usually gives no support according to the motto: It takes two to tango.
- The onset of stress with palpitations, nervousness, headaches, anxiety.
- Chronic state of stress with functional, organic, mental illnesses
- Isolation and loneliness
- In the final stage: rigidity, decompensation, separation or death.

Ermann has aptly put the world of perverse thinking into words:

> Thus, perverse thinking occurs not only in clinically manifest perversion, but can also appear in other mental organizations. It is not tied to either aggressive or sexual acts. Perverse thinking is a functional state that lies outside of reality and the fantasy world and occurs when fundamental change is imminent. It creates a denial as a protection against destruction, but does not actually change reality, but creates a second reality alongside the objective one. It consists of thinking in two incompatible realities at the same time and denying the incompatibility. The coexistence is declared normality. (Ermann 2005, p. 188)

▶ Example

In the last lesson before the Easter holidays, the 8-year-old patient Viel-Wut walks in the door with the words: "Today I'm going to kill you." The psychotherapist Mrs. Hab-Acht is surprised that the patient, after countless sessions of aggressive fantasy games in which murdering and destruction took place, now directs a fantasy directly against her.

She says, "You're mad at me?"

He hisses, " … because you're so insane and always look so stupid."

She ponders and ventures an interpretation, "Maybe you're so mad at me because I'm going on vacation and we can't see each other."

He: "Weirdo, weirdo, weirdo, I don't want to hear any more."

Psychotherapist: "But I came up with it because we usually play well and you've never told me anything like this before."

Him: "I don't want to hear any more, because my anger about the last holiday is not over yet, remember that."

Psychotherapist: "Oh, I didn't know that, ... "

He says, "That's enough," and slaps the table hard.

The psychotherapist reflects. In that the patient wants to "muzzle" her, thus attacking her connection to him, but at the same time his angry reaction has to do with the psychotherapist's vacation and this shows his desire for attachment, she remembers the essay "Attacks on Linking" (Bion 1959), in which Bion describes early closeness-distance conflicts. She decides to attempt a verbal intervention after all because she doesn't want to let the patient go on vacation like this. At the last moment she remembers that the parents had also cancelled (after her) for the Easter holidays because they wanted to go to relatives. She asks the patient, "Are you actually going away for the Easter holidays?" He looks directly at her for the first time in the session, "So what?" (How the psychotherapist then specifically intervened is presented in ► Sect. 6.5). ◄

Example

The couple Problem-Fall had registered because of lustlessness of the husband. In the first session with psychotherapist Bemüht-Sich it becomes clear that this disturbance exists since he became aware that his wife seeks sex in parking lots and saunas. He says that this shocked him and that he also finds it disgusting. He adds that maybe it is unjustified and petty, but he is afraid of disease and that is always in his thoughts when his wife wants sex. The psychotherapist tries hard to put the "symptom" in the right frame by saying that there is a concrete fear that makes it difficult for the man. He shows understanding for the man and for the woman, but shies away from addressing the realism of the fears, instead suggesting that it is important to examine the dynamics of both together, and how they might collude.

To his amazement, they both come to the second session beaming and reporting that all is well. In the first session, the psychotherapist had allayed the man's concerns. They had had intercourse a few times in the past week and he had even managed to avoid using a condom. Mr Bemüht-Sich feels extremely uncomfortable. As he smiles weakly and nods, his mind is racing. He feels that his efforts have been used rather perversely to increase the perverted couple dynamic or scenario of sexuality and degradation and the play of disease and death. And he goes into inner turmoil over the fact that he should also be responsible for it. He feels obligated to point out this dynamic, even at the cost of the couple not coming back. (How the psychotherapist intervened in concrete terms is described in ► Sect. 6.6).

General Strategies to Escape Such a Scenario as a Victim

- Recognition of the mechanisms and one's own powerlessness
- find support
- Act
- Resist internally
- Resist psychologically
- Involve the judiciary
- Expand prevention

5.2.1 Psychotherapeutic Strategies for Mastering a Destructive-perverse Power Game

▪ **1 Help Yourself**

In most cases it is a matter of psychotherapists first having to get themselves out of the danger zone in order to be able to help the other person and themselves from there. Some therapists then have to overcome their own absolute helper role, possibly also the victim role (▶ 2).

In rare cases, when the psychotherapist realizes that he himself is the destructive aggressor, he must protect the patient as soon as possible and seek psychotherapeutic help (▶ 3) or even turn himself in.

▪ **2 Help the Patient Who Is a Victim**

It is often mistakenly said that victims must give up or overcome the desire to suffer. However, this is only the case in rare cases, namely when a masochistic disposition is present. At most, it is a matter of the destructive pervert taking advantage of the victim's masochistic, depressive, or narcissistic part. In most cases, victims are more or less accidentally in the wrong place at the wrong time to become victims of this destructive pervert. Often they do not flee in time, even if they have already recognized how disturbed the person is, and that they themselves are the target of these attacks, because they can see "the good" in the person and think that he or she might change for their sake. The situation is aggravated if the victim has been assigned the role of healer in his or her family of origin from the beginning or has chosen this role himself or herself. Often the victims do not manage alone, among other things a psychotherapy can help. Psychotherapists who want to work with victims of mental and physical violence are advised to actively cultivate communication, to work in a benevolent and activating way, in order to prevent a too abstinent attitude for the patient "not essentially different from the state of affairs which at the time—I mean in childhood—had a sickening effect" (Ferenczi 1933, p. 306). The above-mentioned basic components of the therapeutic attitude are also part of the attitude of mentalization-based psychotherapists.

Likewise, it is helpful not to begin by reflecting on one's own part in the destructive-perverse communication, because the person concerned is already permanently thinking about what he or she has "done again now" and suffers from superfluous feelings of guilt. The alternative would then only be "more of the same" (Watzlawick 1983) and would not lead to any solution.

Psychotherapeutic help can be provided in the following steps:

- Choice of psychotherapist (who is on the side of the patient's goals),
- Calling perversion by its name,
- free yourself,
- free yourself from guilt,
- take a look at your own share,
- Finding your way out of suffering,
- Healing (► Chap. 7).

Or alternatively:

3 Help the Patient Who Is the Aggressor

This group of patients is relatively small. As psychotherapists we mostly deal with the victims. Destructive-perverse people do not often come to psychotherapy because they are not aware of any disorder or unconsciously fear their own psychological breakdown. In order to stabilize themselves, their aggression is directed at the psychic domain of the other person, but in the strictest sense, "mental perversion" does not stem from a psychiatric disorder, but from a "cool rationality combined with an inability to see others as human beings" (Hirigoyen 2002, p. 13). Gruen and Weber (2001) describe that the first interventions must consist of confrontations of these patients with their own weakness, namely their fear and cowardice and specifically their fear of feelings. These interventions easily lead to the discontinuation of therapy in the voluntary outpatient, day hospital or inpatient setting, unless there is sufficient distress for some reason. This may be, for example, that this person has been excluded from their family or group. Exclusion and loneliness is the only thing that reaches these people and can cause self-pity.

Only when confrontations have led to a breakdown of the grandiose and cold defenses can psychotherapy in the normal sense take hold, or can compassion and empathy be allowed and valued. In this respect, influence seems possible, but in treating such disturbance patterns, the practitioner must keep in mind how these patients have grown up. Unlike others, they have experienced no love or a perverse form of love in their early development, they feel fear of love because they do not know how being loved (and loving) feels and affects them.

> In the work with victims as well as with attackers, it must—in the long run—of course not be about a one-sided moral condemnation of the attackers and the approval of the victims, because this maintains the inner-psychic split in the perpetrator-victim system. And the psychotherapist would then join in just as unilaterally as a saviour.

This would prevent the possibility of finding boundaries. Good and elastic boundaries only arise where "good" and "evil" are allowed to unite; in other words, those who are able to delimit themselves have mastered the role of victim. Psychotherapy should therefore be about the integration of parts of the personality that have not been lived. In the long term, it is important to dissolve the inner and outer division into perpetrator-victim, to understand the overall scene and thereby prevent one pole from remaining externalized and continuing to be loved or fought against by projection in the other.

But in all long-term integration efforts it must not be lost sight of that in dealing with destructive-perverse patients the first measures and interventions do not (only) consist in being nice and friendly and showing compassion and the first thoughts cannot go in the direction of integration either, because for this one reaps contempt and is moreover thought to be insecure, unclear and without contours due to the lack of structural preconditions of these patients, and misunderstandings can arise from this. Only when substantive confrontations have led to a questioning of the grandiose and cold defenses can psychotherapy in the normal sense have an effect.

I now turn to the interventions of mentalization-based psychotherapy (MBT), which seem suitable for introducing mentalization as a supplement to the strategies and measures described earlier in this chapter in a narrower sense. Representatives of MBT also treat patients with social behaviour disorders and sociopathic disorders using or involving this approach (Bateman and Fonagy 2008). These treatment approaches are currently being systematically investigated in Germany and are therefore not yet available in manualized form (cf. e.g. Taubner 2008; Taubner et al. 2015).

5.3 Mentalization-Based Interventions

I will present the main features of mentalization-based therapy (MBT) based on the literature of its founders (e.g. Allen and Fonagy 2006; Bateman and Fonagy 2006; Allen et al. 2011). The central aim of MBT is to promote or restore mentalization. The treatment focuses on the attachment relationship between patient and psychotherapist. The psychotherapist always pays attention to a functioning working relationship and tries to ward off attacks on it. Mental processes are observed and encouraged, and in particular attempts are made to identify non-mentalizing processes on the part of the patient and the therapist. This results in the following **general treatment strategies**:

General Action Strategies of MBT

- Provide security, create safe environment—Goal: Deactivate hyperactive attachment system.
- Communicate curiosity, awaken joy, hope—Goal: Activate exploration system
- Promote coherence experience—Goal: Activate identity development
- Generally promote exchange—Goal: Promote mentalization capacity

In order to be able to realize these general treatment strategies, the psychotherapist must be able to recognize the prementalizing modes of thinking described in ► Chap. 2 and take them into account in interventions and formulations. Patients in contingent experience only reproduce what is observable, always appear fragmented. As a psychotherapist, one hardly gets an idea of the patient's everyday world. In the teleological or targeted mode, someone can interpret their own and others' actions as purposive, but cannot discern the causes and motives. Only reality confined to physical space counts, that is, only what can be observed. In the mode of mental equivalence thoughts and external reality cannot be distinguished. The equation word = thought = reality seems valid. Internal states are experienced as real. In the pretend mode, thoughts, motives and fears (as in play) are separated from reality.

Consideration of the patient's mode of thinking also requires a defensive **therapeutic stance**, which is determined by the following assumptions:

- Mistakes do happen,
- not-knowing stance,
- Exploration before insight,
- Process before content,
- Plurality over objectivity,
- Disruption and Recovery.

In each session, the psychotherapist pays attention to which **dimensions of mentalization** can be considered, has the mentalization star (► Sect. 3.3) in mind, if necessary, and tries to loosen fixations or compensate deficits so that a balanced mentalization ability can develop:

- Cognition vs. emotion,
- Self vs. others,
- internal vs. external,
- explicit/controlled vs. implicit/automatic.

The interventions in each session follow the principle that basic interventions such as clarifying, elaborating, confronting and challenging take place on a basis of empathic validation and trust, the viability of which must be repeatedly demonstrated. When these two stages are well mastered, psychotherapist and patient can turn to basic mentalizing, i.e., process-oriented relational experience with exploration of intentions, triggers, and responses is the focus. Then the mentalization of transference can be focused on, whereby the interpretation of transference is not excluded, but is not seen as a goal. In dealing with transference, for example, transference markers are used, projections are not rejected, affects and transference triggers are inquired about, transferences are understood in the patient's reality, and transference content is interpreted. This results in a sequence of foci.

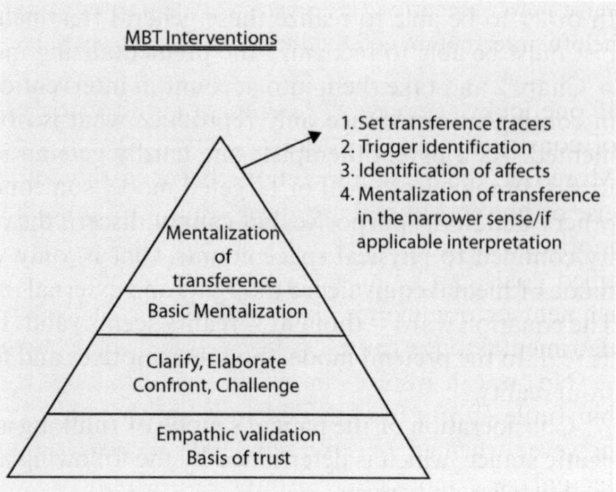

Fig. 5.1 Pyramid of MBT interventions

Sequence of Exploration and Mentalization Foci

- Affects associated with externally observable behavior.
- Emotional and motivational context for affects
- Interpersonal context of affect outside the therapeutic relationship
- The overarching interpersonal theme within therapy
- The specific (transference) context within the therapeutic relationship

In summary, then, interventions are stated to be close to consciousness, or awareness is gradually worked out. "Resistance" is understood as an increased need for joint containing activity within the therapeutic relationship. The therapeutic work takes place step by step, always in interplay with the creation or re-establishment of a secure interpersonal basis in the therapeutic contact (Fig. 5.1).

In ► Chap. 6 I will continue the case vignettes of this chapter, describe interventions of the psychotherapists and examine these example interventions to see whether the respective destructive power entanglement on both sides was successfully coped with. Successful coping does not mean stopping power and influence in their tracks, but rather stepping out of destructive processes, taking into account the ethical and moral principles of the participants as well as empathic responses, and transforming them into constructive processes. First, in ► Sect. 6.1, I will introduce the method of context analysis, with the help of which I analyse the therapeutic processes and assess "successful coping".

References

Allen JG, Fonagy P (2006) Mentalisierungsgestützte Therapie. Klett-Cotta, Stuttgart. 2009

Allen JG, Fonagy P, Bateman AW (2011) Mentalisieren in der psychotherapeutischen Praxis. Klett-Cotta, Stuttgart. 2008

Bateman AW, Fonagy P (2008) Comorbid antisocial and borderline personality disorder and comorbid antisocial personality disorder: mentalization based treatment. J Clin Psychol 64:1–14
Bion WR (1959) Angriffe auf Verbindungen. In: Bott Spillius E (Hrsg) (1990) Melanie Klein heute, Bd 1. Verlag Internationale Psychoanalyse, München, S. 110–139
Dreikurs R (2009) Psychologie im Klassenzimmer. Klett-Cotta, Stuttgart
Ermann M (2005) On perverse thinking. Int Forum Psychoanal 14:188–192
Ferenczi S (1933) Sprachverwirrung zwischen den Erwachsenen und dem Kind. In: Schriften zur Psychoanalyse, Bd 2. Fischer, Frankfurt a.M. 1972
Freud S (1932) Warum Krieg? GW XVI, S. 13–27
Fromm E (1976) Haben oder Sein. Deutsche Verlags-Anstalt, München
Gruen A (2016) Wider die kalte Vernunft. Klett-Cotta, Stuttgart
Gruen A, Weber D (2001) Hass in der Seele. Herder, Freiburg i.B
Hirigoyen MF (2002) Die Masken der Niedertracht. dtv, München
Hurni M, Stoll G (1999) Der Hass auf die Liebe. Psychosozial-Verlag, Gießen
Sandler J (1976) Gegenübertragung und Bereitschaft zur Rollenübernahme. Psyche 30(4):297–305
Taubner S (2008) Entsteht Einsicht im Täter-Opfer-Ausgleich? Eine empirische Studie am Beispiel adoleszenter Gewaltstraftäter. Monatszeitschrift für Kriminologie 91(4):281–294
Taubner S, Sevecke K, Nolte T, Roussow T, Bateman AW (2015) Manual for menalization-based-treatment for conduct-disorder (MBT-CD). Unveröff, Manuskript
Watzlawick P (1983) Anleitung zum Unglücklichsein. Piper, München

How Can I Recognize the Successful Overcoming of a Destructive Power Entanglement?

Contents

M.-L. Althoff, *Mentalizing Power and Powerlessness*,
https://doi.org/10.1007/978-3-662-66119-2_6

Psychotherapy on a clinical level is about keeping an eye on the effects of one's own interventions, especially when one has intervened in a potentially powerful way. When it comes to finding ways out of destructive exercises of power or destructive-perverse scenarios of power and powerlessness, this view of the effects of one's own interventions is indispensable, literally necessary. This chapter begins by introducing the method of context analysis, by means of which it is possible in practice to assess psychotherapeutic interactions and interventions systematically and also "on the fly" as constructive or destructive and then to react accordingly. Subsequently, I will give an exemplary insight into my method of evaluating my own actions by means of context analysis.

6.1 Context Analysis for the Evaluation of Patient-Therapist Interactions

As I have described in detail elsewhere (Althoff 2009, 2013), I work with the context-analytic procedure of adaptive psychoanalysis (e.g. Langs 2004). This procedure will be outlined here again in a basic way. In general, I see my task as a psychotherapist (as well as a supervisor and teaching therapist) as investigating together with patients (and supervisees and analysands) the question of the triple fit, i.e. the fit of patient and therapist as well as the fit of patient and approach (Leuzinger-Bohleber 2001). I also encourage this inquiry when considering the question of dealing with power. As a psychotherapist, can I capture how the patient consciously and unconsciously values the mutual interactions and my interventions? And what value does that have? In working on the patient's unconscious, coded comments, I am guided by the assumption that people have an **unconscious knowledge** of what norms and rules are adequate and beneficial for them and others (cf. Langs 1984; Smith 1991). So I try to identify which interventions are judged by **the patient himself to** be in accordance with his (unconscious) principles and ethics and to contribute to his recovery. How can the unconscious meaning that the patient attaches to an intervention of the therapist (and its implications) be deciphered?

6.1.1 The Context-analytical Approach

The context-analytic approach provides an evaluation concept that provides criteria for the effectiveness of one's work in the ongoing process (in short: "on the fly"). One examines the patient's first derivative reactions after an intervention by the psychotherapist and lists:

- Topics that are positive and affirming or negative and non-affirming; and
- Information that further explains and expands the unconscious insights provided by the intervention that has just been given (cf. Langs 2004). This list is used to assess whether the intervention can be assumed to be validated or falsified (mixed forms also count as falsification).

Langs (1982) gives two criteria for **validation**:

Interpersonal Validation (Langs 1982, 2004)

This means that the patient's reactions express that he or she had an experience of being understood, of good cooperation, of closeness. For example, people who are understanding, wise, kind, supportive, helpful, and memories of valued teachers, a competent doctor, dear friends emerge in the narratives and incidences. Following Stern et al. (2012, p. 258), "vitalization" can be observed. Own studies indicate that there is an increase in the feeling of security (Althoff 2009).

Cognitive Validation (Langs 1982, 2004)

The patient's ideas express that the therapist's regrouping of the material was coherent and opened up new contexts of meaning. It turns out that these new insights are added to the psychotherapist's interpretation. Cognitive validation is represented by narratives that open up new aspects of the patient's symptomatology or resistances, unexpectedly for both patient and therapist (cf. Langs 2004).

In the long term, I also take a complementary look at clinical validation.

Clinical Validation

This is given when the patient's symptoms and relationships improve. In addition, when evaluating interventions in the supervisory relationship, a multidimensional dimension of clinical validation can be considered. This finds "its expression in the benign (...) development of the supervisee's therapeutic interaction with his patient, which can be read off from the patient's (and the supervisee's) unconscious validation" (Kahl-Popp 2010, p. 475).

According to Langs (1982), **non-validation or falsification** is indicated interpersonally and cognitively.

Interpersonally in three ways, namely through

- the absence of narratives or reports or ideas,
- by the absence of positively toned images,
- by negatively tinted themes such as people being blind, uncomprehending, selfish, cognitively by the absence of new, insightful material.

According to the context-analytic method, I am not convinced of the coherence of my intervention until I have received both types of validation from the patient or all three types of validation from the supervisee spontaneously. Non-validating reactions (and mixed forms) make it necessary to reconsider the context and the interpretation, by also including the information received after the intervention.

Concrete Implementation

In the following, as announced, I will continue the examples from ► Chap. 5 and add the interventions of the psychotherapists and reactions of the patients and psychotherapists. In this way I would like to clarify my handling of destructive exercise of power and destructive-perverse power scenarios, at the same time outlining certain recurring conflict situations and illustrating the context-analytical evaluation method. Central to this is the focus on the patient's narratives and experience **immediately following an intervention by the psychotherapist**. This is not trivial or easy, because the therapist's resistance is greatest at that very moment—according to the motto: Who always wants to be measurable? By being in a continuous process of intervention, validation or non-validation, subsequent confirmation or correction, re-intervention, etc., and usually understanding more and more and being able to work together better, validations can become more frequent and profound, and in the long run, through positive introject formation, allow for more symptom-free experiencing and empowering images and narratives.

Step-by-step Explanation of the Procedure and Sequence of the Context Analysis

- **Context: Identification of the Problem Situation and the Context**

Who has shown what kind of exercise of power and when? How did I behave or what did I say? → The starting point is my action, i.e. this is the context (trigger).

- **Processing: Understanding the Patient's Processing, Related to the Context**

Can I put myself in the patient's shoes, do I understand his/her reaction (cognitive and emotional empathy), and can I understand the patient's exercise of power in response to my action?

- **Symptomatology: Concomitant Symptomatology or Resistance**

Has symptomatology or resistance occurred in connection with the problem situation or context?

Intervention: Measures and Interventions

- **Inner Preparation**

Being aware of one's "armoury" or "tool shed"—What do I have at my disposal, e.g. rigour, discipline, ethical principles, moral integrity, resistance to corruption, being able to wield the sword to draw a line, competence, contextual analysis? How do I feel about a silent interpretation, if any?

- **Conducting**

Can I put the acquired understanding into a (verbal) intervention? Is an attitude of assertion and distance or closeness and persuasion more appropriate?

- **Reaction 1: Reaction of the Patient**

What cognitive and emotional spontaneous reactions can I observe?

- **Reaction 2: Own Reaction**

What are my own reactions to my intervention and the patient's reactions?

Evaluation: Evaluation and Decision on Further Action

- **Evaluation**

Were there any validating reactions from the patient and from me? What emotions, images and memories related to the theme of power/powerlessness emerged?

- **Further Procedure**

Are corrections or improvements to my intervention necessary? Then I look for the context that now seems effective to me. Otherwise, I wait until a new context appears (◘ Fig. 6.1).

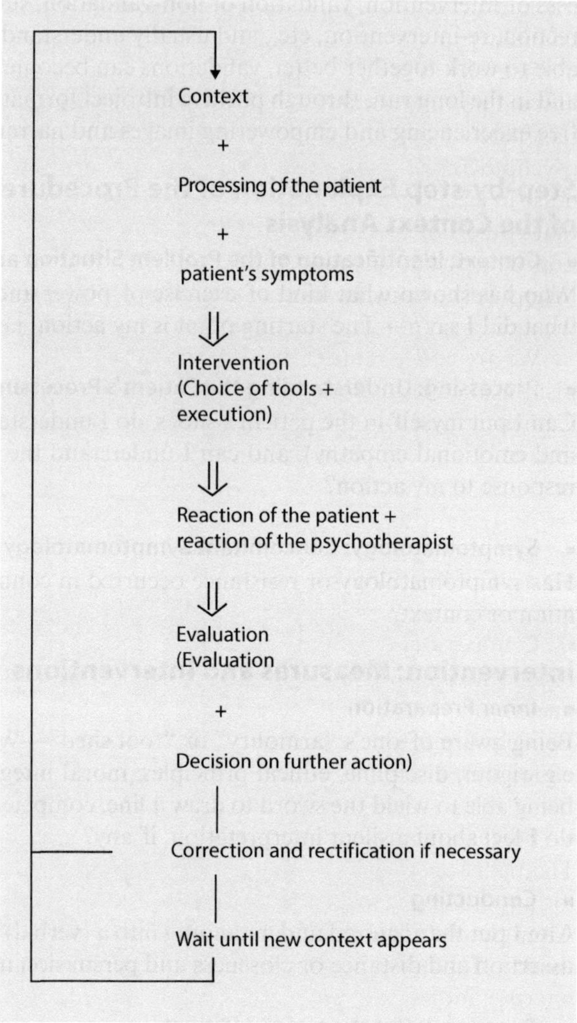

Fig. 6.1 Flow chart of the context analysis

In the next sections I will present the procedure and method as an example with the help of the continuation of the case vignettes from ▶ Chap. 5.

6.2 Overcoming One's Own Destructive Tendencies: Coping with Neurotic Anxiety

I will first continue with the example from ▶ Sect. 5.1.1, first with a summary of what has happened so far: The psychotherapist was surprised that, in his perception, patients were reluctant to be questioned. He assessed himself as precise, factual and logical in his reactions. From self-experience he knows that he sometimes deflects his fear of losing his own identity by feeling similar to others. When there is too much closeness and feeling on the part of a patient, he sometimes tends to ask factually probing questions. In the session under discussion, the patient Vorsicht-Grenze was initially pleased with the empathic understanding, felt close to him, and did not understand why the psychotherapist suddenly became so probing. He remembered situations in which he had experienced his mother as intrusive. The psychotherapist interpreted so quickly that this interpretation, for all its "correctness" in terms of content, was experienced interpersonally as a boundary violation that could not be resolved during the session. The patient left with latent irritation. The psychotherapist first reflected alone, then visited his supervisor Mrs. Hat-Ideen, worked out his anger at himself and his feelings of shame, and waited for the next session.

We are now again the invisible spectators of the next session of psychotherapist Bislang-Sorglos and patient Cautious-Limit. Psychotherapist Bislang-Sorglos is now curious to see whether Mr. Vorsicht-Grenze is still busy with the last session in his unconscious descendants or implicit ideas. We observe the therapist at work.

6.2.1 Context Analysis

- **Context: Identification of the Context**

Psychotherapist Bislang-Sorglos is willing to take his interventions (intrusive questioning and quick interpretation) as context or triggers and see how Patient Vorsicht-Grenze processed them or how the irritability arose and How it then went on for the patient.

- **Processing: Understanding the Patient's Processing**

The patient comes to the next session in good spirits, saying, "Today I am ready for anything; ask what you want to ask, but I will answer when I want to answer. After all, one shouldn't fire any rash shots." The psychotherapist is surprised and thinks, "I didn't expect a reference to the context of "Drilling inquiries and quick interpretations" so "quickly". He waits it out despite a brief flaring impulse to intervene right now, smiling inwardly as he thinks, "I did learn from the last lesson, after all." Patient: "Last week was kind of exhausting. Everyone seems to think that yes, you can do it to me. My boss accused me of not taking good enough care of my clients. And he wouldn't even let me get a word in edgewise. I didn't notice it so much before, but I think he's afraid of getting too involved with my thoughts and problems. Actually, I think he's quite capable, but well, hopefully he'll calm down soon. I'll just back off a bit. Actually, on the whole, everything is fine at my work too, so I can rest easy. But if he's like that with others, he can soon close up shop. Well, maybe that's a bit of an exaggeration."

- **Symptomatology: Concomitant Symptomatology or Resistance**

The patient comes into the session somewhat resistant ("answer when I want to answer"). He indirectly announces that he knows how to resist, with withdrawal and waiting.

Intervention: Measures and Interventions

▪ Inner Preparation

Prepare weapons or tools—He considers which weapons or tools he would like to use or which are probably needed. He realises that the weapons cabinet can remain closed because the patient has not attacked him directly or indirectly. In terms of tools, he estimates that he will be able to use (1) his courage to stand by himself, (2) his ability to recognize contexts in the patient's ideas, and (3) his competence in formulating clarifications and interpretations. "And I may also need (4) controlled self-disclosure," he adds.

▪ Conducting

The psychotherapist now finds that it is time for an interpretation, because the patient has given him enough clues about his unconscious processing of the context, and he has reacted with resistance. Mr. Bislang-Sorglos wants to show that he wants to hold on to the agreement of an empathic and understanding therapeutic relationship. He says: "Mr. Vorsicht-Grenze, I would like to come back to my actions in the last session, because I somehow have the impression that they are still important today, because you said at the beginning today that I could ask what I wanted, that you would answer if you wanted to and would not be tempted to rush to conclusions. I didn't feel comfortable myself afterwards either with asking so many questions and then telling you I was under the impression you were mentioning your mother because I seem so much like her to you." Patient: "My mother isn't that bad." Psychotherapist: "Oh, I can see that. I think now that I can see myself well in your boss asking critical questions but not letting you get a word in edgewise and instead insinuating something, i.e. attacking you unjustifiably. Possibly you have also perceived with me that I am sometimes afraid to concern myself too much with the thoughts and problems of others and thereby lose myself, as it is possibly also with your boss. And then I act according to the motto 'attack is the best defense'. What you are pointing out to me is hugely important, which is that when I am like this, you understandably only see the option for yourself to bide your time, back off and wait for me to calm down (as with your boss). You even tell me that if your boss or I continue to do so, then we could close up shop. In the final analysis, I agree with you. And we both think it won't come to that. But your withdrawal, your defensive attitude, which I have caused, these concern me, because I believe that withdrawal and defensive attitude cloud our relationship and then perhaps bring about a mood of irritability in the two of us or good humour in the separation and being alone. All in all, I should calm down and, we agree, get over my fears."

▪ Reaction 1: Reaction of the Patient

Patient smiles, visibly relaxes: "Well, it's a lot what you hear all day. Where does that leave you with your own thoughts? Sometimes, when I have one appointment after another at the office and so many things of my own on my mind at the same time, I'm afraid of forgetting my private things during the day. And then my wife reminds me a bit rudely in the evening. … I just remembered my mother, but it has nothing to do with you (smiles) … She was sometimes really abusive, but when I think about it, she could have done that out of fears (laughs) … like you … but seriously, I think she was always afraid for me too quickly. I think that's why it's so important to me that I can unfold … Kind of a nice day today. During my session, then often the sun falls in so beautifully … "

- **Reaction 2: Reaction of the Psychotherapist**

The psychotherapist notices that he is relieved and also increasingly relaxed. He can, while the patient is talking, briefly indulge his own thoughts: "Yes, one session at a time; when is it going to be too much; tonight I'm going to think again about my own mental hygiene." He notices that the patient takes steps toward him, jokes with him, and tells him things or suppositions about his mother of which he knew nothing before. The basis of trust seems to have been restored for today. And he registers very clearly how much the patient asks for a "space to unfold". His interpretation and the patient's reaction to it also have a good effect on him emotionally-interpersonally and cognitively.

Evaluation: Evaluation and Decision on Further Action

- **Evaluation**

Overall validating responses emerged from both the patient and the psychotherapist. Positively toned emotions, images, and memories related to the topic of power emerged.

- **Further Procedure**

Corrections or improvements to the interpretation do not seem necessary for the time being. Mr. Bislang-Sorglos waits to see what Mr. Vorsicht-Grenze comes up with next.

6.3 Overcoming a Relationship Dilemma: Getting Out of a Bind

I now come to the continuation of the second example (► Sect. 5.1.2). First of all, I will again summarise what has happened so far: Psychotherapist Verständnis-Gern gave a comparatively large amount of support and encouragement to the self-confident and dependent 19-year-old patient Versorg-Mich. It became clear to her that the patient had always responded positively. However, she did not defer to hints about developmental possibilities. In one session she realized how annoyed she had become with her role as the understanding, caring therapist. She also realized that with this patient she usually talked more than commonly because she was responding to the patient's habit of raising her voice at the end of a sentence.

The psychotherapist was looking for a way to address the situation as simply as possible. Now we again become spectators of the concrete event of the relationship.

6.3.1 Context Analysis

- **Context: Identification of the Context**

For psychotherapist Verständnis-Gern it was clear by now that she had reacted to the raising of the patient's voice at the end of a sentence first unconsciously and finally consciously in response. However, by also being present that she need not have reacted in this way, she became aware that the patient and she had moved as if in a self-reinforcing cycle in which she could be the strong and knowing therapist and the patient could remain the seemingly weak and incapable of action. Unconsciously, however, the patient had exercised power and influenced the therapist through sentence modulation.

6

The psychotherapist chooses as the starting point of her intervention her own responsibility for her role assumption, which is the context, and she takes it upon herself to wait for an appropriate moment.

- **Processing: Understanding the Patient's Processing**

The patient seems tired and says that she has had a headache for two days, not very severe, but it is getting to her in the long run. That's on top of everything else: "You know what I mean," she says, raising her voice slightly. Then she pauses. It is clear that she is now consciously waiting for the psychotherapist to react in the usual way.

- **Symptomatology: Concomitant Symptomatology or Resistance**

The patient complains of headaches and exertion, which may be related to the problem situation in therapy.

Intervention: Measures and Interventions

- **Inner Preparation**

Ready weapons or tools—With this patient the gun cabinet can remain closed, because she would rather be frightened if the psychotherapist would now fiercely and angrily differentiate herself. The psychotherapist reckons that (1) she will need courage to start an intervention, that (2) she should signal a lot of understanding so that the transition to a less caring attitude does not turn out too abruptly, that (3) she should take responsibility for her role assumption, that (4) she should simply intervene so that the patient does not immediately experience herself as incompetent and small again.

- **Conducting**

Mrs. Verständnis-Gern waits a little longer, then summons up all her courage, because the mention of the patient's headaches does not make the beginning any easier for her. At the same time, however, she thinks that the headaches could also be an expression of the fact that they both now feel anger towards each other, she direct anger and the patient turned against herself in the form of somatisation. She says: "Today something occurs to me that is perhaps a little different from what I usually say because it concerns our relationship. It has become clear to me that you just asked indirectly with the raising of your voice if I could think of something about the headaches and the efforts you have had in the last few days. And then I was thinking, I would love to ask you more about when exactly the headache started, if it was after our last session, for example, and what else was so stressful. And then I don't know if I can burden you with that, and I want to address that. It's like a catch-22: If I ask, I may burden you and make you feel weak and insecure. If I don't ask, I'm afraid I'll keep you in the role of the small, insecure, and incompetent, which you profess to not want. Then I would be betraying your goals without your knowledge, and I would feel that I was embarrassing and offending you."

- **Reaction 1: Reaction of the Patient**

The patient spontaneously says, "Wait, I need to think first." A pause occurs. "I think you should ask me if that's what you want. ... That's all I know about it. ... Perhaps you could challenge me more than you do. ... Though I always think it's stupid. For example, my music teacher just called me up and told me to audition. That worked out, not great, but it was a grade B. But he didn't give me the opportunity to talk my way out of it. I thought he was stupid at the time, but that did not seem to bother him , and somehow he made it work with me."

- **Reaction 2: Reaction of the Psychotherapist**

When the patient remains silent, the psychotherapist initially feels quite queasy. She is then surprised at how clearly the patient can draw the interpersonal line ("ask if you want to"). In addition, it becomes clear to her that the patient is telling her, with the reminder of the teacher, that in order to be able to make it with her, one must also sometimes temporarily put up with being found "stupid" by her.

Evaluation: Evaluation and Decision on Further Action

- **Evaluation**

The reactions of both the patient and the psychotherapist are validating. The psychotherapist decides to show the patient that she has understood the last message by laughing and saying: "Then I'll ask if I want to, but you tell me if you think I'm stupid then."

- **Further Procedure**

In the session she waits to see what will happen now. She takes it upon herself personally to reflect once again on her own narcissistic needs to be experienced as helpful and competent in a quiet hour or in supervision or intervision. Overall, however, she is satisfied with the resolution of this relationship development, which was based to a not inconsiderable extent on a mother transference.

6.4 Overcoming a Control-Submission Conflict: Exiting a Power Struggle

The continuation of the third example (► Sect. 5.1.3) begins with a summary of the previous events: The father of a patient, Mr. Nie-Schuld, reported that he often got involved in fights that did not originate from him, although he always tried to fulfil the expectations placed on him. By running quickly into the treatment room at the beginning of the session and being seated by the time the therapist reached the room in an accurate manner, he thus put himself in the listening position, obviously now expecting her to say something. She, however, had refused to speak because she wanted to commit him to the beginning of the conversation in accordance with the agreed basic rule. When she did say something anyway, she believed she was violating the ground rule. She decided to get out of this power struggle. And we watch her try.

6.4.1 Context Analysis

- **Context: Identification of the Context**

Mr. Nie-Schuld unconsciously opened the power struggle in the session by putting himself in the listening position. However, psychotherapist Genau-Genommen suspects that this was preceded by the agreement of the ground rule, which Mr. Nie-Schuld may have felt compelled to do, as a context. To that extent, she wants to see how far she gets by taking her suggestion of the agreement of a ground rule as context.

- **Processing: Understanding the Patient's Processing**

Mr. Nie-Schuld said, "But you've started now." Psychotherapist: "But only because you looked so long." Mr. Nie-Schuld: "Oh, come on, and now it's me again. How did I look?" It seemed as if he was always preoccupied with a question of guilt.

- **Symptomatology: Concomitant Symptomatology or Resistance**

He shows that he is lightly symptomatic or in resistance with his quickness, jumpiness, and mild agitation.

Intervention: Measures and Interventions

- **Inner Preparation**

Ready weapons or tools—She believes that the weapons cabinet can remain closed, but assures herself that she has the key to it in her pocket. She considers which tools she wants to have ready: There is (1) the determination with which she wants to address the power struggle, (2) she wants to keep her wits together in order to be able to justify the proposal of the ground rule well in case of need, and (3) the questioning attitude, and (4) her eagerness to discuss, with which she wants to lead and direct the conversation. For the case of need she (5) also puts the interpretation ready.

- **Conducting**

Mrs. Genau-Genommen is now ready and goes directly to Mr. Nie-Schuld's question: "Yes, I can say something about that. I don't think you're to blame for anything at all, but we kind of just got tangled up. I think there were two rules against each other. One is that whoever looks first is the listener. That's the way it was when you sat down and I came into the room. The other is that I suggested that you start each session telling what came to you." Him: "I had started when I excused my wife." Psychotherapist: "Oh, and you wanted to see if I noticed!" Him: "Exactly!" Psychotherapist: "But then you did have an issue with the beginning. Could it be that you felt torn. On the one hand, you found my suggestion quite reasonable and wanted to fulfill our agreement, but on the other hand, perhaps you experienced it as coercion if it was always to be this way. And that's when you put me in the position of fulfilling the social norm of the 'second looker' after you had already fulfilled your part of the agreement and thought I might not notice. And now I realize that I refused to speak and thus did not fulfill the social rule, and I realize that you challenged me. I know this isn't the most important thing now, but could it be that you also check this in everyday life, whether those who give rules and orders can also hold themselves to something higher, and then there are often entanglements? Anyway, I've been a bit stubborn here."

- **Reaction 1: Reaction of the Patient, Here: Father of the Patient**

Mr. Nie-Schuld smiles: "Respect, you noticed. I actually wanted to see if you'd fall in. No idea why! … It's fun! … I wonder if it's the same in everyday life. It could be. My boss, for example, often parks in a no-parking zone. You don't resent me me, do you?"

- **Reaction 2: Reaction of the Psychotherapist**

The psychotherapist is absolutely amazed at the turn of the conversation and thinks: So that was a relationship test! She smiles inwardly: "I don't like to be told what to do either. But there was no coercion from me. How lucky I was to have my wits about me." On the one hand, she notices that the patient's father likes to discuss and obviously an important topic has been brought up, on the other hand that he is not sure how far he can go with her.

Evaluation: Evaluation and Decision on Further Action

- **Evaluation**

Mr. Nie-Schuld's reactions are mixed and not clearly validating. The psychotherapist also had mixed reactions. Because of the special importance of the topic for the father (and, incidentally, also for the patient), the psychotherapist decided to stay on this topic and not to make it too easy for Mr. Nie-Schuld in order to understand even more background or transference aspects.

- **Further Procedure**

After she is very sure that she does not resent the father for this test, she asks, "What if I resented you?" She is ready to create a new context with this.

6.5 Attacks on Linking: Mastering Through Clarification and Interpretation

I now come to the continuation of the first example from ► Sect. 5.2. I reported that the 8-year-old patient Viel-Wut came to the last lesson before the Easter holidays with the words, "Today I'm going to kill you." Psychotherapist Hab-Acht asked him if he was angry with her. He insulted her and wanted to keep her at a distance, "I don't want to hear any more because my anger about the last holiday is not over, remember that." Mrs. Hab-Acht realized that he wanted to silence her and attacked their mutual connection (Bion 1959). She decided to attempt a verbal intervention because she did not want to let the patient go on vacation like that. At the last moment, out of an intuition, she asked the patient, "Are you actually going away for the Easter holidays?" He looked directly at her for the first time in the session, "So what?"

We are watching to see what happens now.

6.5.1 Context Analysis

- **Context: Identification of the Context**

Although the patient attacks her and wants to silence her, the psychotherapist realizes that this aggression of the patient must somehow be related to the upcoming vacation and the interruption of therapy. So she assumes that the patient is reacting to the context "interruption of therapy due to the therapist's vacation".

- **Processing: Understanding the Patient's Processing**

"Viel-Wut, I think it makes a difference if it's just me not there or if we both go away." Patient (still reluctant): "I'm going with my parents. They didn't ask me." The psychotherapist thinks she understands that the double helplessness causes so much aggression and disappointment in the patient. However, it is also possible that defended grief and fear are guiding.

- **Symptomatology: Accompanying Symptomatology or Resistance**

The aggressive-destructive attitude towards the psychotherapist, the resistance to relationships, the readiness to use violence have a clear symptomatic character.

Intervention: Measures and Interventions

- **Inner Preparation**

Ready weapons or tools: She opens her children's weapons locker and finds in it (1) a Jedi Knight lightsaber, which will allow her to fight with him seriously without hurting him. Furthermore, she takes other tools, namely (2) her courage, bravery, and steadfastness, (3) her love of truth. She wants to use (4) the instrument of clarification and confrontation.

- **Conducting**

"You're mad at me because I didn't ask you if I could go. I guess you also suspect that I didn't want to ask you, that I just wanted to let you know that I was going on vacation. That made you feel so helpless."

- **Reaction 1: Reaction of the Patient**

He sits down and looks at her piercingly, "Will you be back?"

- **Reaction 2: Reaction of the Psychotherapist**

The psychotherapist feels disillusioned and also a little ashamed: does he know that she feels drained and so ready for a holiday that she feels she could go on holiday "forever"? She is touched by the boy's reaction, because of course she wants to see him again despite everything (e.g. his vehemence and aggressiveness).

Evaluation: Evaluation and Decision on Further Action

- **Evaluation**

On the part of the patient and the psychotherapist there are reactions confirming the bond, i.e. emotionally validating. In addition, the patient's question as to whether the psychotherapist would come back clearly extends her understanding, because until then she had thought he was angry because of the helplessness he had experienced, his fear had not become clear to her (mutual cognitive validation). She told him, "You know, I'm in desperate need of rest, and maybe you and I can have a nice vacation, and I'll be glad to see you again after the holidays. I'll look up when our next appointment is."

- **Further Procedure**

The psychotherapist is attuned to the fact that the subject of fear of loss and rejection is far from being laid to rest. But she is waiting now and is curious to see what will show up after the holidays or with what issues the patient will come back from the holidays.

6.6 Overcoming Perverse Object Use: Exit Through Clarity and Confrontation

Finally, I come to the second example in ▶ Sect. 5.2: The couple Problem-Fall had registered because of the husband's listlessness, which had existed since he was informed that his wife sought sex in parking lots and saunas. The psychotherapist Bemüht-Sich took pains to name the "symptom" as not being an incomprehensible reaction on the part of the husband. He showed understanding for both spouses, but shied away from including the immediate reality, i.e., the real risk of infection and disease from unprotected sex.

At the beginning of the next session, Mr. Bemüht-Sich felt extremely uncomfortable when the couple reported that he had allayed the husband's concerns and they had had sex a few times. He wondered why his efforts had been received so counterintuitively, so that it might seem that his intervention had been woven into the perverted couple dynamic or scenario of sexuality and degradation and the play of illness and death. He decided to address this suspected dynamic, taking the risk that the couple would not return.

We'll watch him succeed.

6.6.1 Context Analysis

6.6.2 Context: Identification of the Context

The psychotherapist undoubtedly feels taken in, spun into the dynamics of the couple and, worst of all, (consciously) misinterpreted. Nevertheless, he has to admit to himself that he had been too unclear in the session before and had confronted the couple too little with reality. Therefore, the only possible context for him is his own lack of clarity.

- **Processing: Understanding the Processing of the Patient, Here: The Couple**

Husband: "You've helped us so much already. I don't know when we haven't had sex this good." Wife: "I wouldn't have expected that. After all, people often say of therapists that they're not so modern." The psychotherapist's interventions have been used at will by the couple, with (conscious) acceptance of twisting and perverting the meaning of the interventions in the process.

- **Symptomatology: Concomitant Symptomatology or Resistance**

Mr. Bemüht-Sich understands the couple's reactions, including being intimate with each other again after the previous session, and their comments at the beginning of the current session, as highly symptomatic. He also judges the attempt to use this to weave him into their problem as pathological. However, it should be noted that the couple does not feel any pressure to suffer or initially has no awareness of the symptom value of the behaviour.

Intervention: Measures and Interventions

- **Inner Preparation**

Ready Weapons or Tools – In this case, Mr. Bemüht-Sich is ready to open his weapons cabinet to put out (1) the sword with which he can draw a clear line. Then he additionally recalls the tools of (1) discipline and (2) integrity as well as (3) clarity and (4) confrontation.

- **Conducting**

Mr. Bemüht-Sich needs to sort. "Not so modern" seems to him a gross distortion of the facts. In more recent times, he feels that there has been rather an increase in the awareness of contagion dangers in sexual intercourse, and he does not even feel that he is at the forefront of this movement. He feels a great reluctance to approach the couple and contact them now. He thinks that this may be a similar aversion to what the husband had previously reported in relation to intimate contact with his wife. He disciplines himself because he feels obligated to point out the bias and fulfill his responsibility of a clear statement. He says, "I have the impression that last time you didn't understand me in the way I meant it. I think I may not have made myself clear. Besides the fact that I think we should understand what drives you, Mrs. Problem-Fall, to have sex with others and what you, Mr. Problem-Fall, then think and do and how you react inwardly, I would like to state clearly that it is a risky thing to arrange to have sex with strangers unprotected. Was I not clear enough there, or was it a maneuver on your part to get me involved in your game so that your relationship could intensify over the past week?"

- **Reaction 1: Reaction of the Patient, Here: The Couple**

They both look at Mr. Bemüht-Sich for a moment. The first thing the man says is something like, "I think you're making yourself clear now." His wife says, "But actually, it was clear last time that he didn't like it. He just didn't say it clearly. Probably wanted to be polite." The man: "Politeness won't get you far. Isn't it always said that politeness comes before a fall?" The woman: "You've got that mixed up, that was the pride. But we can get on with it now. You said something about momentum last time." Man: "And now we listen carefully."

- **Reaction 2: Reaction of the Psychotherapist**

He doesn't care what happens. The main thing is that he made his point. It feels like being rescued from great danger. He's amazed that the patients want to stay. And he realizes that the couple offers so much in quick succession that he can't even process it.

Evaluation: Evaluation and Decision on Further Action

- **Evaluation**

Both the couple and the therapist have validating reactions to the psychotherapist's specific intervention. It is probably astonishing for both that for the first time someone from the outside dares to address a perverse maneuver of the couple.

- **Further Procedure**

They are interested in further sessions. How far psychotherapy can lead is uncertain. Mr. Bemüht-Sich does not consider corrections or improvements of his intervention necessary. He takes it upon himself to go through the session again step by step, e.g. the man's blunder ("politeness comes before the fall") does not leave him alone. Spontaneously, he thinks, "Too much politeness can bring me down in working with this couple."

The method of context analysis entails that interventions in situations of the exercise of power, i.e. in situations that have to do with the subject of power and in which influence is exercised, simultaneously produce emotional reactions, inner images and memories that are associated with power. The psychotherapist relates these reactions, images and memories to the context that he himself has set. In this way, he relates himself to the topic of power and indicates which way of dealing with power he himself understands as constructive or destructive, or which evaluation he has taken from the patient's expressions. Through the subsequent process of evaluation in therapy, psychotherapist and patient then exchange views on the topic directly and personally and not only in relation to others and in an abstract way.

If it has been possible to recognize destructive exercise of power, to understand it and—if necessary—to get out of it, to cope with it and to initiate transformation processes, it usually goes—either one after the other or in parallel—into a longer phase of working through and healing as well as setting the course in the outside. This phase often begins with the exchange of inner images.

References

Althoff ML (2009) Der Sichere Rahmen. Peter Lang, Frankfurt a.M

Althoff ML (2013) Die vakante Sitzung in Psychoanalyse und Supervision. Forum Psychoanal 29:139–160

Bion WR (1959) Angriffe auf Verbindungen. In: Bott Spillius E (Hrsg) (1990) Melanie Klein heute, Bd 1. Verlag Internationale Psychoanalyse, München, S. 110–139

Kahl-Popp J (2010) Kontextanalytische Supervision in der psychoanalytischen Ausbildung. Psychotherapeut 55:471–476

Langs RJ (1982) Psychotherapy: A Basic Text. Jason Aronson, New York

Langs RJ (1984) Die Angst vor validen Deutungen und vor einem festen Rahmen. Forum Psychoanal 5: 1–18 (1989). Original: Making interpretations and securing the frame. Int J Psychoanal 10:3–23

Langs RJ (2004) Fundamentals of adaptive psychotherapy and counselling. Palgrave, New York

Leuzinger-Bohleber M (2001) Katamnesen – ihre klinische Relevanz. In: Leuzinger-Bohleber M, Beutel M (eds) Stuhr U. Langzeit-Psychotherapie. Perspektiven für Therapeuten und Wissenschaftler. Kohlhammer, Stuttgart

Smith DL (1991) Hidden conversations. Routledge, London

Stern D et al (2012) Veränderungsprozesse. Psychosozial-Verlag, Gießen

Working Through and Healing: Dealing with Powerlessness and Manifesting Power

Contents

M.-L. Althoff, *Mentalizing Power and Powerlessness*,
https://doi.org/10.1007/978-3-662-66119-2_7

After overcoming a situation of destructive use of power, there is usually a longer phase of working through, in which inner images of power and powerlessness are processed, in which the constructive handling of power is expanded in a mentalizing way, and in which the question of how power can manifest itself in the patient's life is pursued. Patients and psychotherapists can then work out what—internally and externally—can be changed, what must be endured or, to use Nietzsche's phrase, what is not only to be accepted and endured but willed as fate. It is illuminated how psychological injuries heal, how regeneration and convalescence can be initiated. In conclusion, it is suggested that as a psychotherapist, following resolution from a power entanglement, one should always ask oneself whether or not one is using the "power of circumstance" in an appropriate way with one's way of framing and handling.

In the phase of working through and healing, the method of context analysis (Sect. 6.1) and the elements of mentalization-based therapy (Sect. 5.3) can usefully continue to be consulted and applied. The founders of MBT have emphasized that the reference to mentalization is not bound to a certain psychotherapy direction or certain methods:

> We boldly assert that mentalizing—paying close attention to and reflecting on one's own mental state and the mental state of others—is the fundamental common factor of psychotherapeutic treatments. (Allen et al. 2011, p. 21)

I myself apply context analysis and elements of MBT in the various psychodynamic, depth psychological and analytic settings and in every process phase of my practical work.

The phase of working through and healing is not characterized by the fact that other issues and conflicts cannot also become important or urgent here, because many parallel processes are constantly running, of which sometimes one and sometimes the other is in the foreground of the experience and processing. In this respect, I am now concentrating in an ideal-typical way on the phase of working through and healing after a power entaglement, although I am aware that in practice other processes will usually be going on at the same time. Furthermore, I am aware that the issues in this chapter are only outlined in a rudimentary way due to capacity constraints.

In the phase of working through and healing in relation to a mastered and overcome power vs. powerlessness dynamic, patient and psychotherapist can extend the constructive handling of power and powerlessness into all mentalization dimensions (Sect. 3.3) in a mentalizing way, e.g. by:

▪ Working Through (Inside)

Patient and psychotherapist can work through the inner images of power and powerlessness that emerge.

▪ Working Through (Emotional)

Patient and psychotherapist can identify experiences of power and powerlessness from deeper layers and early experiences.

- **Working Through (Cognitive)**

Patient and psychotherapist can recognize that which can be changed and that which must be endured or, to speak with Nietzsche, that which is not only to be accepted and endured but to be willed as fate.

- **Working Through (Outside)**

Patient and psychotherapist can reflect on how power can manifest itself concretely in life.

- **Healing (Self)**

Patient and psychotherapist can look for ways and means to heal old psychological injuries.

- **Healing (Other)**

Patient and psychotherapist can search for ways to enable lasting solutions from destructive power and powerlessness entanglements.

- **Healing (Explicit)**

In addition, sometimes very concrete, small exercises are helpful, to which the patient is guided. New skills need to be practiced. Then one uses the power of practice, but also experiences mistakes and setbacks. A mistake-friendliness should be practiced, being careful not to make the same mistakes over and over again. Some of these exercises are presented here.

- **Healing (Implicit)**

Mostly it happens that patients spontaneously have their own ideas about which exercises and healing methods could be helpful and then try them out with pleasure.

- **Set the Course**

The psychotherapist may ask himself or herself whether he or she is still satisfied with his or her general frame handling or whether he or she should reconsider his or her own principles of the relationship between frame handling and the exercise of power, the use of the power of circumstances.

7.1 Working Through: The First Questions

Regardless of the initial situation in which patients find themselves, whether they have recognized or not recognized destructive use of power in their lives to date in its full scope, whether they know or do not know why they persevere in their life situation at all costs or find themselves in such a constellation again or relapse for the umpteenth time, most ask themselves in one form or another at some point the questions "Why didn't I get out immediately?", "Why me of all people?" and "Why is this happening to me?". Of course, there is a very individual answer for each patient, which must be found together.

7.1.1 Why Did I Not Get Out Immediately?

I would like to name a few patterns here that prevent those affected from leaving a destructive relationship immediately or from getting into it in the first place.

■ **The Usual Destructive Scenario**
Some already know destructive entanglements from their own childhood. It was lived by the parents or other caregivers, so it is (was) normal at first. At some point they start to consciously suffer and feel pain. They may also get an idea that there are other relationships and partnerships.

■ **The Experience of Meaninglessness**
Life without the beloved partner seems pointless. The partner has no ambition to want to change anything permanently. Separation talks are everyday life, but without effects or solutions.

■ **Xenophobia**
Active struggle would bring with it threatening consequences which the attacked person feels unable to bear. Separation is also out of the question, e.g. for fear of social decline, loss of reputation, loss of material security.

■ **Fear of the Future**
It is often heard that those affected believe that they will never be able to love someone like this again, or that they will never find someone again. It feels like everything will be over. These feelings are usually stronger and more long-lasting if the person has never lived alone before or if it is the first firm partnership.

■ **Low Self-esteem**
Those affected cannot imagine that they could be worthy of being loved for their own sake, because of their personality. Already the experiences in their childhood and youth have brought them to this conviction. They often compensate by sacrificing themselves for their partner. They feel needed and loved for what they give and feel it is normal to receive little themselves.

■ **Co-dependency and Anxiety**
Affected persons who are trapped in co-dependency experience (unconsciously) intense fear and terror in the face of the danger of losing the partner and being alone. The destructive behaviours of the partner are repeatedly excused to themselves and also to others with new explanations.

■ **Co-dependency and Helper Syndrome**
Some remain anchored in a helper role, even when they have long realised that somehow it cannot go on like this. This happens all the more easily if they were already given this role in childhood or had taken it on. They want to understand their partner, therefore excuse their destructive behaviour and want to save their partner or help him or her, even if they themselves go down in the process.

Adapted Behaviour

Those affected have been brought up to conform. They have internalized that important caregivers or even everyone else is always right. Then the destructive behavior of the partner remains unquestioned, without evaluation and without consequences. Often the relationship gets into a destructive spiral because no limits are set for the other person and thus feedback is missing.

Bullying in Youth

Some of those affected have not experienced destructive exercise of power in the form of exclusion and bullying in their parental home, but as young people in their peer group. Such experiences can also promote a permanently conformist attitude and contribute to the fact that the person always does right by everyone else.

Fear of Failure

Those affected cannot give up, but feel obliged to make their partner see reason. They hope they can make it, not give up, not fail. They feel that they have managed to do everything in their life—so why not this? They are then more likely to fight outsiders who ask why they aren't doing anything. They may then become aggressive, withdrawn, depressed or obnoxious towards others, children, parents, friends, colleagues.

Overlooking of Mental Health Problems

Many do not realize until late in life what situation they are in, which usually means that they have already suffered enormously (unconsciously), physically and psychologically and are debilitated. Depression, psychosomatic complaints or addictive behavior overshadow the partnership. At some point, even the regeneration and high phases are no longer of any use, the affected person realizes that they will end up again more and more quickly in exhaustion, helplessness and feelings of inferiority. Fearing their own collapse, those affected soon realistically no longer trust themselves to do anything. There is no longer enough strength to break away and start a new life.

Addictive Behavior

The pretext is usually that they need their partner, that they cannot be without him or her. Over time, it becomes increasingly clear that those affected do not want to be alone, according to the motto: Better a destructive partnership than none. In severe cases, this can be an expression of relationship addiction, and this is independent of the current destructive partnership.

Resistance to Change

Some do not want any changes because they are otherwise satisfied with everything, with the material situation, the environment, the family situation. Then those may think that they leave everything as it is because of the children. It is sometimes not easy to distinguish life lies from reasonable arguments and a double life from a reasonable transitional solution.

7.1.2 Why Me?

This is a question that is relatively easy to answer, but one that is sometimes difficult for those involved to face. If the relationship is severely destructive, the partner will also have admired something about the other, but this admiration is usually reduced to a factual statement. It is told, for example, as a "dry factual report" (Hurni u. Stoll 1999, p. 49):

> We were both interns, a bit isolated and homesick. One day we decided to invite two secretaries from the company to dinner. One of them became my wife. Why her? It's very simple. The other intern was tall, and I'm short. The colleague took the other secretary, who is ten inches taller than my wife. (Eiguer 1989, quoted from Hurni and Stoll 1999, p. 50)

It is more or less a coincidence that the person concerned entered the life of the aggressor at the time when he or she was looking for someone who could confirm him or her and whom he or she could also admire. Admiration, however, usually means that the person consciously or unconsciously has the impression that he or she can make good use of the particular skills, strengths, or zest for life, that they "look good on him or her." He or she is not looking for a personal exchange, but wants the affirmation of a person whom he or she admires but is expected to conform in everything. The person was simply in the right place at the right time or in the wrong place at the wrong time, depending on his or her point of view. That is all.

7.1.3 Why is This Happening to Me?

It should be pointed out once again that working on one's own part must not be the first and certainly not the only measure in working on a destructive connection. As a rule, the first step is to encourage the attacked person to take on less responsibility for the trauma:

> Coming out of one's sense of guilt allows one to reappropriate one's suffering, and only later, when the suffering is far away, when one has had the experience of healing, can one come back to one's personal history and try to understand why one got into this destructive connection, why one did not know how to defend oneself. For one must live to be able to answer such questions. (Hirigoyen 2002, p. 224)

However, if it seems appropriate, the patterns, the unconscious pathogenic beliefs and conflicts that have led those concerned into a destructive relationship and kept them there can be examined, recognised and worked on. It is clear that those who have not recognised in time where their own boundaries lie, that they have not managed to gain respect, that they do not have sufficient self-determination mechanisms, right from the start. But it is central to then clarify what the underlying dynamics are. This part of psychotherapeutic work is not the focus of this chapter. Therefore, I now move on to the next question.

7.1.4 Why Did I Want to Have This Experience?

When those affected have left the destructive relationship **somewhat intact or intact again,** and have gained some clarity about why this happened to them, then the way is usually free to see this experience as an opportunity for further development. What opportunity for further development has been presented to me? What wants/ wanted to be resolved? There are as many answers to this as there are individuals. What all answers have in common is that patterns or conflicts from the past or present have been activated and are pushing for a solution out of suffering or that a new (life) perspective is to emerge that cannot be based on what has been there so far. If the person can see himself or herself as an actor, then he or she can ask the question, "What do I want this experience for?" This question implies that the person accepts his or her fate, or more to the point, as Nietzsche puts it, wants his or her fate. This basic attitude towards life, namely wanting to master life, is postulated in theories such as the Control-Mastery Theory as an early driver of development from early childhood (see, e.g., Weiss 1993; Albani et al. 1999).

7.1.5 Exercises: "Acceptance" and "Letting Go"

The major goal that I believe needs to be addressed in order for power to manifest itself concretely in the lives of those affected is the acceptance of sole responsibility:

- No one can concretely help them set boundaries because it is their boundaries that they only feel themselves.
- No one can concretely help them get respect because they only know themselves when they want respect.
- No one can concretely help them with self-determination, because only they know what they want to decide for themselves.

This big goal does not reach itself and cannot be achieved in one step. Rather, it is necessary for those affected to first take many small steps—if necessary together with the psychotherapist. I propose here two exercises from the abundance of possible exercises.

> As a psychotherapist, you should be creative here and always see which exercises seem suitable to you, which fit the respective patient and do not represent an excessive demand.

Exercise: "Acceptance"

Start by accepting the things in this world that are the way they are. Things which have always been this way, which you cannot change. This may sound easy, but it could be the hardest thing in the world. Can you emotionally and rationally accept the following ten facts? I think it's easier to accept individual concerns and problems if you can first do it with the facts that generally apply. We can discuss these points and see what feelings arise.

Ten Facts that Can Be Discussed

1. You will eventually have to say goodbye to all your friends and loved ones.
2. You're gonna die.
3. The problems never stop.
4. Your past is gone.
5. You can accept your circumstances and change them if necessary.
6. People are different.
7. Not everyone believes what you believe.
8. There is love and hate in this world.
9. People will judge you or what you do as they see fit.
10. You will have to make difficult decisions and live with the consequences.

What do you think of that line:

> One is in our power, the other is not. In our power are: Accepting and perceiving, wanting to act, desiring and rejecting—everything that we ourselves set in motion and are responsible for. Not in our power are: our body, our possessions, our social standing, our position—in short: everything that we ourselves do not initiate and are not responsible for. (Epictet 2004)

Exercise: "Letting go"

Bring the feeling, the thought, the person, the relationship into your body as an image that you want to let go of. Feel it, don't push it aside. Where do you feel it?

Step 1: Can You Stand and Accept the Feeling?

Feel the feelings and thoughts that come. Can you accept this feeling, thought or memory? It doesn't matter if you answer yes, no or something else. The main thing is to wait until an answer arises on its own.

Step 2: Can You Accept Everything that Shows up in Connection with it?

Can you accept whatever has come forward with this feeling, your thoughts or memories? If there are impulses to want to push the feeling away or change it, accept that urge or need as well, if you can. Then again wait for the answer to the question: can I hold and accept all thoughts and feelings and memories and also this urge? Yes, no or anything else, it doesn't matter.

Step 3: Can You Let Go of All that?

Can you let go of all that now? Yes, no, it doesn't matter what the inner answer is. If the answer is yes, ask yourself: When will I be ready? When can I let go of all this? If the answer is no or undetermined, you can go through the questions again if you like. We'll then start again with step 1. And again, there are no right or wrong answers. It just takes time.

Through these questions you may slowly open up more and more inside.

Please don't try to change the feelings or push them aside. Maybe they will dissolve. Just try to be there and accept everything. We can go through the questions again if you think it's not enough.

7.2 Working Through: The Power of Words, Images, Myths and Fairy Tales

7.2.1 The Power of Words

The conversation has a special significance in psychotherapy. Therefore, the verbal communication skills of psychotherapists receive special training and supervision during their training. Psychotherapy is known to expect change and healing of the patient to a large extent through the power of words. This usually includes the accompanying gestures, facial expressions, intonation, etc., which can reinforce, neutralize, or weaken words, and also form a significant part of the effect of words. Words can have a positive or negative impact, they can build up and destroy, they can help, comfort and heal, but they can also discourage, offend and sicken. Thus, the words with which a diagnosis is communicated can trigger very different reactions in the patient. It may be that the patient loses all hope or finally sees a perspective again. In talking to the patient, the psychotherapist may boost confidence in the patient's self-esteem and self-confidence, or he may lower and unsettle the patient's confidence in himself. But it is not only the words exchanged in the conversation between the patient and the psychotherapist that are important, but also the inner dialogue that each person has with himself. The inner dialogue determines the emotional state, the attitude towards oneself and others, and conversely the inner dialogue is determined by the patient's beliefs and attitudes. The psychotherapist has an influence on the patient's inner dialogue through the way he conducts the conversation. He can create inner images through his words and thus work on the inner patterns and, if necessary, try to change them. Likewise, the patient's words can also evoke familiar or new images in the psychotherapist and supplement or correct his or her view of things.

Moreover, we are all familiar with the fact that with our words alone we can bring beautiful, moving, sad or terrible images, stories, myths and fairy tales to life in ourselves and others. Working on inner images is the central task of psychotherapists:

> Therapists try to put other people in a position to call up inner images that offer security when fear-producing images threaten to become overpowering and thus determine thinking and action. And they try to open up again, to dissolve, to make wider and looser inner images that have become too narrow and overpowering and that lead a person's thinking, feeling and acting into increasingly narrow dead ends. (Hüther 2006, p. 16)

7.2.2 The Power of Inner Images

Inner images can emerge in the patient, for example, after interventions by the psychotherapist or after his or her own actions. But they can also be actively stimulated by the psychotherapist. According to Hüther (2006), inner images are the ideas that we carry within us and that determine our thinking, feeling and acting. They can be thought of as patterns stored in the brain that we need to find our way in the world. These images are helpful in planning actions, facing challenges, and responding to threats.

> As far back as we can even think, people have apparently developed inner images about the nature of their external world and used them to shape that world. (ibid., p. 11)

In his book "Prinzip Menschlichkeit" (Principle of Humanity), Bauers writes about the power that emanates from images of people (Bauers 2007). They shape how we deal with the world and what we expect from it. Sometimes it just needs to be one person in a child's life who is good to them and shows them that they themselves matter. Hüther (2006), for example, mentions the case of a man who relates that he moved from ward to ward in the kinship and then from home to home over several years.

> When I was ten years old, I met a teacher in one of these homes. (…) He was the first person I had met until then who really looked at me (…). (…) It was (…) so that (…) learning (…) now all of a sudden started to be really fun for me. (…) I started to read a lot and suddenly found everything in these books incredibly exciting. (...) After half a year (…) I had other teachers again, but I didn't lose my desire to learn again. Somehow I have carried the image of this one, decisive teacher with me ever since. (Hüther 2006, p. 106f.)

Faced with ever more realistic images and films, even animated films, our perception of external reality becomes ever clearer, more detailed and sometimes overpowering. The world of our inner images is in danger of being paid too little attention, of being over-formed by the ideas of others (e.g. the media), of being considered small and unworthy in comparison, and of slipping into the unknown and unused for lack of attention. In this context, we can only go new and individual ways if we orient ourselves according to our own, creative ideas and not according to mass images and canned images: "It is high time to think about the power of our inner images" (ibid., p. 13).

A special opportunity is offered by the processing of images that emerge in connection with the processing of a power/powerlessness issue. What image emerges in the patient when he or she thinks of anger, e.g. triggered by a situation inside or outside therapy or triggered by an intervention of the psychotherapist, e.g. the angry father, the angry mother, the cold father, the cold mother? And what does the psychotherapist remind you of when he or she has made an intervention? Do I even seem human to the patient anymore, you sometimes have to ask yourself as a psychotherapist. Sometimes they are traumatic memories, and the "involuntary and unbidden memories form a kind of repetition of the trauma" (Hirigoyen 2002, p. 226f.). In this book I do not go into specific methods of trauma treatment, because that would be a topic in itself (cf. on this, for example, Reddemann 2001 or Spangenberg 2014).

Verena Kast has also become known in therapy through the method of Active Imagination developed by C.G. Jung. The aim of the method is that dominion and sovereignty over tormenting thoughts and images is gained by patients learning to encounter and deal with them. Kast (1988) gives the example of a woman who experienced in her fantasies a figure that looked like a judge. This figure constantly reproached her for everything she had done wrong in life. The inner figure said, for example, "You have messed up your life!". In therapy it was important to critically deal with this destructive figure, the judge, with the help of Active Imagination. The aim was to free the patient from her self-destructive authority complex by initiating a critical attitude of consciousness, so that a healthy self-esteem could grow (cf. Kast 1988, p. 191ff.).

The question for the psychotherapist is from which of the three levels of consciousness the patient's powerlessness to be dealt with originates (Sect. 3.2). Is it time to consciously address this powerlessness

- to bear,
- to endure,
- to convert,
- to disagree,
- to defy the law,
- to overcome,
- differently and to act alternatively,
- differently by alternative defense strategies?

What images of power and powerlessness do you carry within you? These images are also (unconsciously) powerful for your patients. If you like, do this little exercise in four steps. Have a blank sheet of paper and a pen ready and read step by step:

- **Step 1**

Close your eyes. Feel it breathing inside you! Take three deep breaths. What image comes when you think the word "power". Memorize the image well … Describe or paint the image!

- **Step 2**

Close your eyes. Feel it breathing inside you! Take three deep breaths. What image comes when you think the word "powerlessness". Memorize the image well … Describe or paint the image!

- **Step 3**

Close your eyes. Feel it breathing inside you! Take three deep breaths. What image comes when you think the word "My power". Memorize the image well … Describe or paint the image!

- **Step 4**

Close your eyes. Feel it breathing inside you! Take three deep breaths. What image comes when you think the word "my powerlessness". Memorize the image well … Describe or paint the image!

Were these unexpected images? What did they trigger? Do you want to work with these images or revise these images, perhaps in conversation with colleagues, friends, supervisors, self-experiencing guides? When I was at the beginning of intensively working with the themes of power and powerlessness and did this exercise, unexpected, frightening images emerged in each of Steps 1 and 2. The image for power was that of the Minotaur and the image for powerlessness was a hospital bed. In the meantime, these images have changed.

7.2.3 The Power of Myths

A myth is a narrative with which people and cultures express their understanding of the world and themselves. In religious myths, people's existence is linked to the world of the gods. A myth is difficult to grasp in its meaning. In our time it also seems that myths are less often consciously told, shared and interpreted. For example, before the image of the Minotaur came to my ownmind, I would not have thought that this myth played a major role in my inner unconscious life. It is possible that myths unconsciously play a more significant role in everyone's life than we think possible.

Joseph Campbell (1994) has written extensively on the subject of the power of myths. He thinks that people created their culture with myths, that even the first images, i.e. the images on cave walls that have survived to this day, were magical in nature. They said something about how people saw themselves. The first words that were written down referred to the gods and created the word myth that has been handed down to us.

The myth of Theseus, for example, tells the story of the Greek hero Theseus. He had set himself the task of defeating the Minotaur, a creature with a human body and a bull's head, in the labyrinth of Crete. No longer should seven Athenian maidens and young men have to be delivered to him every nine years. This was a most dangerous undertaking, for Theseus had to go into the labyrinthine cave to do it, find the Minotaur, defeat him, and come out of the labyrinth again. He killed the monster and with the help of the king's daughter Ariadne—who had given him a long thread—was able to find his way out of the labyrinth.

The myth of Theseus is often interpreted as a representation of the confrontation with one's own, as yet unrecognized (aggressive) drives, which a person, especially a young person, has to face. A myth allows for many interpretations, always says only between the lines what the parable might be for someone, but it is precisely in this that its fascination, effectiveness and orienting power is seen. Instead of always looking at everyday life and everyday worries, it seems to be a need and a help for many people to be able to recognize, understand and orientate their own life in a larger pattern. In our culture there is a need for the activation of the inner hero and heroine, as Campbell (1994) and Zimbardo (2007), for example, suggest.

> A myth from which culture develops is to be distinguished from an **artificially introduced political myth** as a stereotyped and controlled image of history, which entails great dangers. This artificially created myth is intended to emphasize in the collective memory what a particular party or ideology considers necessary.

National Socialism, for example, was such a political movement, because not only were jobs and collective cohesion promised, but this movement also wanted to be a "sense-making" movement of great myths, symbols and rituals. An artificial mythology was concocted from various elements, transfiguring heroes of the past into patterns of identification for the present. A searching, aggrieved people was promised spiritual orientation and the establishment of a "millennial empire" reaching into eternity. For example, an "Aryan" myth of origin was created, which was supposed to define the superiority of the Germanic peoples over all others. Even today, mythology is used in the right-wing scene to lend justification and plausibility to völkisch racist world views.

7.2.4 The Power of Fairy Tales

The magic and secret message of fairy tales transport us to a bygone world of "once upon a time". Fairy tales tell stories that may seem outdated and cruel today. Behind the manifest story, in the depths of symbolic meaning lies its true treasure (e.g., Fromm 1981; Kast 1983, 1984; Ermann 2005). Children intuitively grasp the high value of fairy tales; they cannot get enough of some. The tales can make them suspect that despite all the sorrow, hardships, blows of fate, and problems they experience, life can still hold a path that allows them to be happy and content. It is believed that fairy tales were told to pass on important intuitive knowledge about human beings to the next generation (Langs 1996). They were not primarily intended to entertain children with funny or scary stories, but it can be assumed that the teller usually had intuitive knowledge about humans and translated this knowledge into images and stories to pass it on.

When working with fairy tales in psychotherapies, an understanding of the many small symbolic clues can draw attention to the messages of the fairy tales. Whoever has developed an understanding of these symbolism and messages, the manifest action is no longer so much in the foreground, i.e. it is not so important, for example, whether the witch is burned or imprisoned for life. The only thing that is important then is the actual message behind the action, which may have fascinated and unconsciously preoccupied the patient even as a child.

7.2.5 Exercises: "Inner Source" and "Favourite Fairy Tale"

When it comes to healing from destructive power entanglements, it often means "being able to reconnect the scattered pieces, to close the circle" (Hirigoyen 2002, p. 227). The patient and psychotherapist can work together to find ways to heal old psychological injuries. For example, they can "learn to protect their autonomy, to avoid verbal violence, to reject attacks on their self-esteem. The person is not 'globally' masochistic, but the pervert has tied him up because of his weak spot, which may be a masochistic one" (ibid., p. 228). Only when this realization has been gained can the patient and psychotherapist seek ways to facilitate lasting solutions from destructive entanglements of power and powerlessness.

The following two exercises are small steps that patients can take when a blockage has been released, when something has "flowed" internally. Being able to draw from their own "inner source" connects patients, for example, with their inner strength and creativity. Even the simplest meditation exercises can have a great effect, such as the well-known power exercise "Inner Source".

- **Exercise: "Inner Source"**

Imagine flowing water ... in which direction does it flow? ... follow the water against the direction of flow ... go on and on until you come to the source ... the water is clear and cold and refreshing ... it is your and only your source, which is inexhaustible.

- **Exercise: "Favorite Fairy Tales"**

What was your favorite childhood fairy tale? Please tell me! What fascinated you most about the story, the main character, the other characters?

7.3 Healing: The Cold Heart: From the Loss of Feelings

The fairy tale "The Cold Heart" is a well-known fairy tale by the early deceased storyteller Wilhelm Hauff. The hero of this fairy tale, Peter Munk (called Kohlenmunk-Peter), wants to be more than he is and sells his heart to a messenger of evil, the Dutchman-Michel, who sells the wood from the Black Forest expensively in Holland. Peter Munk persists in a state of self-alienation by gambling, dancing, drinking, and striving for wealth and outward prominence. The turnaround occurs through a change in his inner attitude and evaluative standards with the help of Tannhäuser's glass man, who granted him one more respite. Peter manages the turnaround in a symbolic seven days. Peter and his wife Lisbeth find their way back to each other and have a child, and his mother can return.

Symbolizing the power of money as the sole end purpose and the loss of feelings is the cold heart of stone that makes rich and remains cold when the poor lament. This concept of the ultimate end can be found in Simmel (1900, p. 358), who writes:

> For even such goods that are not in themselves of an economic nature, money, having become a final end, does not allow them to exist as definite values coordinated to it; it is not enough for it to set itself up next to wisdom and art, next to personal importance and strength, yes, next to beauty and love, as a further final end of life, but in doing this it gains the power to degrade those others to means for itself.

Meanwhile, many people, and not only pronounced narcissists, suffer from fear and greed at the same time. Their relationships are characterized by coldness, self-interest and lack of empathy. Wolfgang Schmidbauer (2011) states that the consumer society lacks emotional maturity and that the modern money economy works against people's feelings and empathy. Homo consumens (Fromm 1976), the cold-hearted consumer of the planet, is doomed to extinction like the dinosaur once was. The cold heart arises from fear and powerlessness and feeds on it, on massive fear,

- to be overrun by feelings, to no longer be able to control them and to drown in this flood,
- drowning in grief and pain,
- to sink into the bottomless pit and lose your footing,
- to suddenly become aware of oneself in one´s own helplessness.

Thus, as long as possible, people try to emphasize the special and to live even more consumer-oriented immoderateness, at the price of moving even further away from their own emotional world. Thus, possibly—similar to the fairy tale of the coal-munk Peter—the rediscovery of empathy on various levels becomes the only chance of salvation for Homo sapiens.

7.3.1 Exercise: "Getting Into Feelings"

At first it is best to choose comparatively mild situations and feelings. When you have felt and described these first feelings, we turn to larger tasks.

Describe the feelings that arise at the thought or memory of

- a work colleague you like,
- a nice TV movie,
- having a nice summer day,
- a lovely party,
- a rainy day,
- a disappointing meal at a restaurant,
- a missed meeting,
- a piece of clothing that didn't come in your size.

7.4 Healing: The Bleeding Heart: About the Powerlessness of Melancholy

The opposite of the stony heart is the bleeding heart, which makes poor and bleeds out when the poor lament and at the same time it has become cold or deaf to its own hardships and needs. To recognize more precisely the special mental risks of the helping professions—this concerns patients from helping professions and psychotherapists themselves—is important, sometimes necessary in the truest sense of the word, not least for psycho-hygienic reasons. The often deeply rooted helper attitude is a major cause of burn-out, the "burning out" of once committed and competent helpers. In addition, helping people who are or have been exposed to severe traumatic stress involves many risks of its own. Pross (2009) describes how psychotherapists and teams of helpers who are confronted with the most severe suffering and disturbance in crisis regions, after natural disasters or even in therapeutic practice can reach their limits.

The fairy tale of the Sterntaler tells the story of a poor orphan who has nothing but a piece of bread. She goes out into the world and on the way gives away her bread, her cap, her bodice, her skirt and finally her shirt. Then the stars fall as gold coins from the night sky (symbol of spiritual power), and she has a new, fine linen shirt on in which she can collect them. Among other things, this fairy tale gives the message that it is important for givers to also be able to receive and use resources. It is important to always keep a watchful eye on this ability.

7.4.1 Exercise: "Receiving"

Imagine the circle of your loved ones or draw it. Now, in your mind or out loud, give each one "Three things I love about you". Feel what you are saying.

End the circle by telling yourself three things you love about yourself.

And when you do this exercise with your loved ones in reality, feel what they say to you.

7.5 The Relationship Between Framework Management and the Exercise of Power

After overcoming a power issue, resolving a power entanglement or uncovering one's own destructive use of power, every psychotherapist should ask himself or herself whether one's own frame handling fits the newly gained knowledge about the use of power or whether he or she should fundamentally change something about it. After all, frame design and handling indicate whether one is using the power of circumstances in a beneficial or in a destructive way. This now brings us back to the level of everyday basic psychotherapeutic action.

7.5.1 Framework Components: Harnessing the Power of Circumstances

Why do we actually design a framework the way we do? You might spontaneously think: We do what we think is right. But if we think about it a little longer, we might notice that the connection between ethical principles, our convictions and our actions is by far not as close as we initially believe. Let me illustrate this with an example from everyday life: people often eat "unhealthier" than they "really" want to. We exercise less than we had planned. We spend less time with family and friends. In short: our real behaviour is often far removed from our convictions, ideals and principles. Now you might think that we are all just too weak. We all know situations in which the "inner bastard" is used as an allegory for our own weakness of will. However, I believe that the framework components of our private and professional lives, as well as the framework conditions of society and politics, have a much greater influence on our behaviour than we are normally aware of.

Let us look at an example from everyday life: Let's assume psychotherapist Reist-Gern is on a long journey, for example to the Lindau Psychotherapy Weeks, and gets hungry. She has long resolved to eat "healthier", but today she does not have enough food and drink with her for such a long journey. Drinks are usually not a problem, as water and tea are on sale everywhere. But food: as a car traveller she stops somewhere at a petrol station or bakery or she goes to the on-board bistro (train) and chooses something from what is on offer. To that extent, what is available also has a strong influence on her actions, possibly as strong an influence as her good intentions. It is clear that no one, not even our Mrs. Reist-Gern, is forced to eat unhealthily. After all, she could have brought more from home. It would have been more inconvenient, but it could have been done. So the general conditions alone cannot be the sole reason or justification.

If we look more closely, we realize that the problem is that we don't usually have just one goal. Mrs. Reist-Gern, for example, has not only the resolution to eat healthy, but also the goal to spend little time preparing for a trip, not to have such heavy luggage and not to lose so much time when traveling. As a rule, we can't optimize all of our goals, and there is rarely one goal whose optimization we subordinate to all others. In the end, goal optimization is always a pragmatic trade-off between optimizing a variety of different goals, given the constraints of the situation at hand. In concrete terms, this means that if Mrs. Reist-Gern is "suddenly and unexpectedly" hungry on her trip, she tries to satisfy this need without losing sight of her other goals. So she goes to a bakery or the on-board bistro and chooses from what is available. She could endure the hunger, or she could interrupt the journey and go in search of a fruit and vegetable shop, but if she does not do this, it is not out of convenience, but because she would then give lower priority to other goals, e.g. arriving in time for the meeting, in a good mood and full.

This is where the power of the framework comes into play: whether in the bakery or on the train or any vendor, we choose from what is available. It rarely happens that one finds an offer so unacceptable that one rejects it and takes nothing at all. Who always crafts a greeting card when the stationery shop's offer didn't include the exact card. This means: the given offer has a very big influence on our behaviour. And we are not protected from suggestion and influence either. It influences our choice in which position (in view or hidden) and how attractively (as "offer of the week" or "our classic") the alternatives are presented. Mrs. Reist-Gern's gaze, for example, first falls on the sign "Offer Belgian sugar waffle" together with a "hot drink", and she only discovers the "Bircher muesli" later.

In this respect we choose, but always only from the current offer. We do not choose "freely", but move within the framework that is set for us by the available offer. Often we do not even notice this consciously or we accept the framework as fixed and hardly influenceable. In this respect, we choose bound by the alternatives available and by the time and energy—and bound also by the amount of energy we are willing to spend on it in view of other goals and tasks.

Many years ago, for example, I was looking for practice rooms to rent. At the time, the supply was small, the premises on offer seemed far from ideal, and my pipe dreams of having a separate entrance and exit door, for example, receded into the distant future. Of course, I would have had the opportunity to invest more time and energy to create a more attractive alternative. I could have waited, could have extended my search spatially, could have considered buying or building a practice property, but at the cost of thereby having even less time for other goals and then therefore being forced there more to make a pragmatic choice from the alternatives given. And so it is with many tasks: The important ones and the less important ones, the ones that are in the center of our attention and the ones that are not consciously paid attention to, all tasks have to be covered and done somehow, but they are not all equally important to us or do not all have such a high priority that we are willing to accept greater sacrifices of other goals or pay the necessary price for them. Often we act under time pressure and out of pragmatism in the more or less clear awareness that what we are currently doing or how we are doing it does not "actually" correspond to our goals and good intentions, but we also know that anything else would be more strenuous, more time-consuming and, on top of that, would be associated with noticeable disadvantages elsewhere. So we may choose not to engage in a provisioning fee dispute again because it seems too strenuous and risky (Althoff 2013).

It follows from these considerations that one could actually dispense with the constant subliminal guilty conscience from which many people suffer in view of these constant compromises, in favour of a conscious and reflective consideration of the available alternatives. Instead of punishing oneself with a guilty conscience for the inevitable compromises, it is healthier and wiser, for example

- to accept that compromise is always imperfect,
- to ensure that there is a fundamental awareness of the trade-offs involved in decision-making,
- to pay attention to which compromises run counter to one's own priorities,
- to realize that in the case of constant overriding of health and private life, a guilty conscience does not help, but only a course correction,
- to recognise that a compromise that has been agreed but is not viable may well cause a guilty conscience, but that it is more important to make the best of the situation,
- to consider that our role in a power development sometimes makes us feel bad, but that after overcoming this entanglement only a course correction related to the framework handling and personal development is helpful.

7.5.2 Against the Unreflective Adoption of Frame Components

As much as we sometimes suffer from the "lazy" compromises of everyday professional and private life, it seems to have proven practical in life to focus on the alternatives that are available and not to be constantly preoccupied with possibilities that might be better but are not available. At the same time, however, this expedient behavior makes us susceptible to unthinkingly and unconsciously accepting the defaults given by circumstances. We then think within the given framework without being aware of the power we thereby grant to circumstances.

▶ **Example**

Psychotherapist Druckvoll tends to take higher risks when he is under deadline pressure, e.g. exceeding speed limits when he has left home too late, or neglecting annoying side tasks, e.g. postponing documentation until the weekend, or being worse at setting limits, e.g. squeezing even more appointments into an already full week. Sometimes he is upset with himself for putting others' health and his own at risk over an appointment, whatever it is, and is already inviting further pressure for the future. In quiet moments he realizes that under the pressure of deadlines or circumstances he does not even notice how his boundaries shift and how the framework conditions then change his actions, although his convictions and ideals remain the same. ◀

Presumably, Germans have a higher average retirement pension compared to Americans, not because they place a higher importance on it than Americans do, but because in Germany a fixed percentage of income is automatically contributed to the statutory pension scheme. If it were an active choice for Germans how much they wanted to set aside for retirement, they would probably pay in drastically less overnight.

In my opinion, the example of occupational disability insurance provides evidence that our personal old-age provision has little to do with a typically German need for security. Few Germans have one, even though it covers an existential risk and even though occupational disability insurance probably makes as much sense as pension insurance. It is the same with the decision to have psychotherapy. Fewer Americans seek long-term psychotherapy not because they oppose it or don't need it, but because, unlike Germans, they can't count on their health insurers—if they are members of any—to cover the costs. Presumably, many people tend either to postpone difficult decisions for the time being or to choose the recommended option in each case. This applies to old-age provision, occupational disability insurance and—often just as risky—approving of licence agreements and installing software, where most customers accept the default.

Even with things that are actually important to us, we adapt to the given circumstances, with the danger that these circumstances never change. Circumstances are rarely such that they favour long-term goals even in the short or medium term. While Ms. Reist-Gern's goal is to eat healthier, there are no spelt biscuits at gas stations in the short term, and in the medium term she will not be able to cook clear soup and make salad all the time during the Lindau psychotherapy weeks. And possibly, when she returns home, she will find that her refrigerator is empty and there is only one frozen pizza left in the freezer—unless Mr. Reis-Gern has done the shopping and already prepared everything fresh and delicious.

Often we cannot prevent the short and medium term goals from taking over. Before we completely run the risk in everyday life that the exception becomes the rule and we usually take the path of least resistance, we can set "alarm clocks" for ourselves and become attentive when it might be worthwhile, for example, in the short term to choose a little

- more complicated,
- more unusual,
- more troublesome,
- strenuous.

An "alarm clock" can be, for example, to make an agreement with oneself that one consciously realizes that something is going wrong right now, when one wants to cancel the regular sport for the second time, when one wants to push a supernumerary appointment into the calendar for the second time, etc., and to take countermeasures.

Conversely, this tendency towards the path of least resistance means that for us as providers, decision-makers or leaders, in order to achieve changes in behaviour, we don't need to approach changing people's attitudes and beliefs so much. Rather, it is important to change the framework (or the offer) so that a different behavior becomes meaningful from their subjective perspective in order to achieve their goals. The usual effort, I think, is the other way around: we often think that we need to convince other people first so that they can see a different behavior as meaningful and necessary. But first, we can only change ourselves, and words alone can often do little to shake people's beliefs. Secondly, even if a change in beliefs were successful, there would be no guarantee that it would then actually result in a change in behaviour and then in the desired way. In this respect, I think that if you want to persuade someone to change their behaviour, you should look at what you yourself can change for the better, i.e. concentrate on changing your own attitude and the framework conditions. Ultimately, this is always the result of a context analysis. This knowledge results in a special responsibility of the individual, but also of the employer, the state, the provider.

> If you want people to make the most sensible choice possible, then you should preset that choice, because most people will choose that preset, implicitly recommended solution.

Some economists say that only wisely set standards could reduce old-age poverty, poor nutrition, energy waste. Moreover, it will then be possible to dispense with pressure and coercion. No one will be able or want to prescribe a healthy diet, but if the menu of the day at the rest stop or in the on-board bistro is healthy, eye-catchingly presented and reasonably priced, more people will probably opt for it, and Mrs Reist-Gern would be pleased.

By the way, as a consumer, it is not very effective to try to change the views and goals of corporations, rulers and suppliers by expressing opinions and publicly criticizing them. It makes more sense to change one's own consumption behaviour and to influence others to do the same.

For the therapeutic context it could be formulated like this: Wherever symptomatology appears, it is worthwhile to reflect on the context or the framework components that one has set oneself. How can the patient's behaviour or symptomatology be understood? As caused or facilitated by the "power of circumstances"? How could a more conducive environment be created by changing framework components? What framework components make it (unconsciously) meaningful for the patient to behave in exactly this way? Often, a better understanding of the framework and the patient's reactions to it is key to understanding the patient's behavior and difficulties while initiating positive clinical development. That this explicit reflection on the framework components and thus the "power of circumstances" is by no means trivial is impressively demonstrated, for example, by Zimbardo (2007) in his book "The Lucifer Effect—The Power of Circumstances and the Psychology of Evil".

▶ Example

A middle-aged patient has come for her first interview. Encouraged by the analyst's initial question, she begins to talk about the reason for her coming and her biography, and talks and talks and talks.

Analyst Mr. Angestrengt listens, takes in what is being said, holds back, occasionally gives a "Hm" as a sign of his presence, moves from time to time—all in the spirit of the frame component of neutrality. He observes his countertransference, which at first consists in a feeling of being overwhelmed, then his ears buzz, he can no longer think of a word, his empathy no longer seems to work. He interprets his countertransference as a reaction to an intrusive relational intake. Nor does the patient respond to a clearing of his throat or an insistent look, but continues. As the session draws to a close, the patient is unable to answer the question of what she wants to achieve with the therapy, for she says: "You must know that. I've told you everything now, haven't I?" To which he says, "Not like that." She says, "Okay, then don't." And leaves.

Analyst Mr. Mühelos has a similar countertransference. He decides to become more active and to implement the framework component of neutrality in the sense of the attitude of consistently siding with the patient's goals (Control-Mastery Method, MBT). He says, "Yes, and then?" and interrupts her when it becomes too much for him or he no longer understands anything. The patient is visibly disturbed, but his interruptions change her behavior. She gives shorter answers. She continues to report; he listens and interrupts when he tires; she gives answers. It does not become a joyful interaction, but at least a rudimentary two-way conversation. He doesn't know if the treatment can succeed, because the brief moments when he allowed the intense counter-transference were violent. But they agree to talk again.

A small change in the frame component of neutrality changes the outcome of the initial interview: Analyst Angestrengt engaged in a power/powerlessness play, with a destructive outcome, while Analyst Mühelos also engaged in his countertransference, but countered it in favor of a more conducive mentalization-based relational design, thus enabling the relationship. ◀

Overall, then, the importance of attitudes and beliefs for practical action should neither be overestimated nor underestimated. The word "actually" very often indicates that we act differently than it "actually" corresponds to our values and beliefs. But by this we do not mean that our attitudes and beliefs are unimportant to us and should simply be ignored. Let me use the example of speeding again. When you get a fine for speeding, it usually makes a big difference whether you were "flashed" in a spot where you can understand the speed limit or not. While many people are moderately annoyed when they receive a fine for a speed limit they can understand, the reaction is much more severe when the speed limit seems arbitrary. This can even go so far that the fine is paid, but the perceived arbitrariness leaves hatred and hostility towards "those up there".

At the same time, however, one should not underestimate the importance of attitudes and beliefs. There is an absolute necessity to make the frame conditions set comprehensible if one cannot or does not want to enforce them in a rough way (Althoff 2009, 2013). Especially when changes strongly interfere with the patients' scope of action, their consent and agreement strongly depend on whether these changes are comprehensible to the patients or seem arbitrary. Even if attitudes and beliefs are usually not sufficient to change behavior, they play an important role as catalysts of change.

If one has recognized the "power of the frame conditions", one will therefore know that persuasion is not superfluous. It does, however, take on a different status. One will not expect attitudes and beliefs to trigger change, but will expect them to play a determining role in the acceptance of change. Persuasion is then a factual task in the therapeutic process that can stimulate the patient to become aware of his or her opinions, attitudes, evaluations, and perspectives for change. Beyond the concrete psychotherapeutic situation, knowledge of the importance of the power of circumstances can also contribute on a larger scale to changing social conditions.

References

Albani C, Blaser G, Geyer M, Kächele H (1999) Die "Control-Mastery" Theorie—eine kognitiv orientierte psychoanalytische Behandlungstheorie von Joseph Weiss. Forum Psychoanal 15:224–236

Allen JG, Fonagy P, Bateman AW (2011) Mentalisieren in der psychotherapeutischen Praxis. Klett-Cotta, Stuttgart. 2008

Althoff ML (2009) Der Sichere Rahmen. Peter Lang, Frankfurt a.M

Althoff ML (2013) Die vakante Sitzung in Psychoanalyse und Supervision. Forum Psychoanal 29:139–160

Bauers J (2007) Prinzip Menschlichkeit. Warum wir von Natur aus kooperieren, Hoffmann und Campe, Hamburg

Campbell J (1994) Die Kraft der Mythen. Artemis & Winkler, Zürich

Eiguer A (1989) Le pervers narcissique et son complice. Dunod, Paris

Epictet (2004) Handbüchlein der Moral. Reclam, Ditzingen

Ermann M (2005) On perverse thinking. Int Forum Psychoanal 14:188–192

Fromm E (1976) Haben oder Sein. Deutsche Verlags-Anstalt, München

Fromm E (1981) Märchen. Rowohlt, Reinbek b. Hamburg, Mythen, Träume

Hirigoyen MF (2002) Die Masken der Niedertracht. dtv, München

Hüther G (2006) Die Macht der inneren Bilder. Vandenhoeck & Ruprecht, Göttingen

Hurni M, Stoll G (1999) Der Hass auf die Liebe. Psychosozial-Verlag, Gießen

Kast V (1983) Mann und Frau im Märchen. Eine psychologische Deutung, Walter, Olten

Kast V (1984) Familienkonflikte im Märchen. Eine psychologische Deutung, Walter, Olten

Kast V (1988) Imagination als Raum der Freiheit. Walter, Olten

Langs RJ (1996) The evolution of the emotion-processing mind. With an introduction to mental darwinism. Karnac Books, London

Pross C (2009) Verletzte Helfer. Klett-Cotta, Stuttgart

Reddemann L (2001) Imagination als heilsame Kraft. Klett-Cotta, Stuttgart

Schmidbauer W (2011) Das kalte Herz. Von der Macht des Geldes und dem Verlust der Gefühle. Murmann, Hamburg
Simmel G (1900) Philosophie des Geldes. Anaconda. Köln. 2009
Spangenberg E (2014) Behutsame Trauma-Integration (TRIMB). Klett-Cotta, Stuttgart
Weiss J (1993) How psychotherapy works. Guilford Press, New York
Zimbardo PH (2007) Der Luzifer-Effekt. Spektrum-Verlag, Heidelberg. 2008

The Social Dimension

Contents

M.-L. Althoff, *Mentalizing Power and Powerlessness*,
https://doi.org/10.1007/978-3-662-66119-2_8

This concluding chapter deals with the dimension of the topic outside the direct patient-therapist relationship. The changed way of dealing with power and powerlessness should in the best case be able to bring about a change and improvement for the patient in his or her life and also prove to be a meaningful enrichment for the psychotherapist in both professional and private life. Otherwise, one could move in an ideal dream or pretend world, which is unconsciously carried by the common idea "If only the world were different, then we would have it better", which—certainly exaggeratedly formulated—could then be called a "folie à deux".

Just as in the individual, personal, professional and private context, the change of one's own attitude and the framework conditions can also be seen as an instrument of social change. For a changed attitude, together with a meaningful design and change of framework conditions, can also be of determining importance for desired social changes. This view of things seems to me to be more necessary than ever in view of the news about the finiteness of resources, climate change, terror and the danger of nuclear war. For at the same time, Internet communication at the speed of light makes us all neighbors. Lipton and Bhaerman (2009), for example, are convinced that everything can change for the better and that by changing our beliefs we can influence the "spontaneous evolution" of our species and thus shape a more enjoyable future. If this were to succeed, it would mean that a large proportion of people would learn to use the "power of circumstances" and not feel trapped in powerlessness.

8.1 The Professional Policy Dimension

In Germany, we are currently experiencing in the field of psychotherapy that work is being done at the level of professional policy to change the framework conditions of care and training through the planning of a new Psychotherapists Act, which could fundamentally change the current form of care and training. The psychotherapists who are active in the care of patients and in the training of psychotherapists are hardly ever consulted about what changes the majority of them consider necessary and sensible. The future framework conditions are negotiated at a higher level rather than relying on grassroots persuasion. And once a change has been decided and implemented, all those working at grassroots level will (have to) align their work with it.

8.1.1 The Development of Guideline Psychotherapy in Figures

The introduction of guideline psychotherapy into the statutory health insurance system in 1967 has had a lasting influence on the development of psychotherapy in Germany. The numerically strong dynamics are reflected in the data assembled in ◘ Table 8.1 on the basis of statistical data from the National Association of Statutory Health Insurance, which can be found in the commentary Psychotherapy Guidelines (Rüger et al. 2015).

Table 8.1 Increase in the number of psychotherapists (1980–2010)

Year	Number of psychotherapists in Germany
1980	1600 medical psychotherapists 550 psychological psychotherapists and 430 child and youth psychotherapists 3526 medical psychotherapists 2211 psychological psychotherapists 682 child and youth psychotherapists
1998 (immediately before the adoption of the Psychotherapists Act)	8571 medical psychotherapists 7997 psychological psychotherapists and child and youth psychotherapists
2010	5420 medical psychotherapists working exclusively or predominantly in psychotherapy (total of all physicians qualified to provide standard therapy 11,652) About 13,801 psychological psychotherapists About 3507 child and adolescent psychotherapists

This development resembles a triumphant advance of guideline psychotherapy, with which, after all, it was achieved that every insured citizen has a right to the assumption of costs of psychotherapy with correspondingly given indication and that every psychotherapist has a certain protection against the forfeiture of fees. Nevertheless, one should be aware that guideline psychotherapy has come to shape our conception of psychotherapy. This can be exemplified by a small detail: Almost nobody thinks anymore about the cases in which it is actually indicated to take a complete anamnesis and diagnosis at the beginning of a treatment process. Every psychotherapist knows that anamnesis and diagnostics are necessary in order to be able to write the report to the expert for the application for psychotherapy. I do not object here to the fact that the anamnesis and diagnostic phase take place, I only plead for remaining aware of the setting of the course through the power of circumstances or the framework conditions.

8.1.2 The Peer Review Process

The necessity of quality assurance is prescribed in the Social Code for all areas of statutory health insurance. Currently, I consider the application and expert procedure according to the psychotherapy guidelines and agreements to be the best of the quality assurance instruments available. Of course, it has to be discussed in which area and on which level quality should and can be assured. The application procedure and especially the report writing are undeniably burdensome, but the procedure protects psychotherapists through (relatively) clear conditions, because

- by delving into the case, the psychotherapist obtains clarity,
- the expert review process ensures the continued existence of psychotherapy as a statutory health insurance benefit,

- every psychotherapist knows when and to what extent therapy can be provided,
- after approval by the health insurance company, the approved sessions are certain,
- no interruption or change can be ordered by the health insurance fund,
- Therapists may not be taken into recourse, e.g. if the therapy has not brought about a change.

I am not arguing here for the retention of the expert procedure at any price and for all eternity, but only for it to be retained as a tried and tested procedure until something better, which protects the individual in the same way, is found. With this, I would like to express my hope that the game of professional politics will be played out as appropriately as possible.

8.2 The Social Dimension

The dynamics of power that play out within a therapeutic relationship and also on the professional-political stage are, of course, reflected in similar scenarios on the larger economic and political stage. I do not want to claim here, in a trivial equation, that the therapeutic working alliance—entered into by mutual consent—is directly comparable to the large and complex events around societal or global agreements and alliances. There are merely a few phenomena on both the small and the large stage that I would like to name in this concluding chapter, and dangers that I would like to point out.

8.2.1 The Dynamics of Narcissism and Power

At every turn in power politics, one encounters the dilemma that access to power and its exercise—despite all rational considerations of the transience of power—inevitably nourish fantasies of greatness, invulnerability, and grandiosity, while conversely, these very fantasies foster the unconditional careerism and ruthlessness that pave the way to the control centers of power. In other words, economic and social power exerts an irresistible pull on people in need of strong narcissistic validation.

In extreme cases, these people are even narcissistically disturbed, and due to this disorder they can realize, for example, an uncompromising career addiction, ruthless self-centeredness, winner-loser mentality and lack of compassion, which opens the way to economic or political power for them. It is well known that these people thus seek to compensate for their (unconscious) feelings of deep powerlessness, helplessness and inferiority. In addition, narcissistically disturbed leaders usually only allow promoters, yes-men and admirers and those who are particularly good at telling others what they want to hear, regardless of their personal opinion, into their vicinity, so that they also create a constant confirmation of their self-image on the outside. This makes a realistic self-perception even more difficult, and illusions and enemy images can become entrenched. In the introduction to his book

"Narcissism and Power", Wirth (2002) already summarises that the narcissistically disturbed person—blinded by his own fantasies of grandeur—loses contact with social reality and must ultimately fail. In my experience, the loss of reality then favours a slow increase in a "suitable" environment: loss of reality, turning away from one's own norms, values and ideals, obsession with power, vindictiveness, ruthlessness, cynicism, brutality, exploitation, contempt for people.

There is such a thing as succeeded narcissism, that is, "true" self-love. This healthy narcissism is characterized by a usually relatively balanced mental equilibrium. Of course, this does not mean that the person is always free of negative actions, e.g. behaving selfishly, using other people, using power in relationships, having grandiose fantasies from time to time, being reckless, envious, jealous, seeking revenge, in short: living out the dark side. But through this attraction of one's own shadow side there is the danger of either having to split it off rigorously and project it, e.g. onto the "morbid and perverted narcissists" in power "up there", or to succumb to the seductions and not to act on the upper level oneself, but to become the stirrup holder of "actually" rejected machinations.

▪ The Narcissistic Personality

People who "suffer" from pathological narcissistic personality disorder are notable for an unusual degree of self-centeredness in their interactions with others, as well as their strong need to be loved and admired by others. Also found at the same time is an inflated self-concept and a seemingly excessive need for validation from others. The emotional life is shallowly developed, and there is little empathy for the feelings of others. If you look closely, you will also notice that they have little joy in life. They seem restless and are easily bored, making longer in-depth conversations almost impossible. A narcissistically disturbed personality is often driven by mistrust and quickly has the feeling of having been devalued or humiliated. The usually underlying unconscious feeling of shame becomes a corrosive poison that releases fantasies of revenge and retaliation.

Most often, narcissistic personalities behave in a parasitic and exploitative way in their relationships with other people. They have no sense that they have other people at their disposal without any feelings of guilt, in order to drop them "like a squeezed lemon" the moment they no longer need them (Kernberg). They act according to the motto: "Better to reign in Hell than serve in Heaven" ("Paradise Lost", John Milton, 1667).

It is also known that these people like to surround themselves with intelligent, rich, powerful or beautiful people whom they can adorn and use to extend their power, but they are not allowed to question them. The narcissistically disturbed person, although uncompromising in their own expressions of criticism, is absolutely hypersensitive to any criticism or refusal. Then, if anyone who is in a relationship with this person wishes to remove himself or herself from the influence, he or she is rigorously expelled. This goes so far that he is denied any right to exist. He then no longer exists, definitively according to the motto: If you are not for me, then you are against me, and then I no longer need you. This is, for example, something that normal relationship partners neither understand nor believe they can bear. The loss of reality can escalate to the point where the ruthlessness, cynicism and contempt for humanity reach levels that are unthinkable for normal people. All this works only because narcissistic personalities manage, to a puzzling and astonishing degree, to protect themselves from the painful feelings in relationships by keeping themselves inwardly out of everything. Rigidity, imperturbability, untouchability (when others have already been deeply shaken) are the greatest obstacles to successful psychotherapeutic treatment of narcissistically disturbed personalities. If they engaged in treatment, they would have to allow pain and depression, and subjectively they would initially feel more miserable than before. Basically, this mental illness consists in the inability to be sick and weak, the inability to suffer, to grieve, to feel fear and to admit one's own weaknesses—a paradox from which it is difficult to find a way out.

In my opinion, it is so important to be aware of these structures and one's own position, because narcissism and power play a role in the life of every individual. Such conflicts can play a role at every level of social interaction, in families, friendships, communities, in professional life, in political engagement. Overwhelmingly, there seems to be an opinion that unfairness and unfair attacks are a problem of free enterprise and high power politics. This opinion could be a consequence of business openly emphasizing the importance of strategy and persuasion and competition. However, research (Copray 2010) suggests that the phenomenon is even more common in public service, social and church organisations. But this is not easy for some to believe, because it would destroy illusions. We all bear responsibility in our environment for the fact that narcissistic disorders must not simply be acted out, because they poison relationships at all levels, they hurt, have a destructive and disintegrating effect, and can kill people.

8.2.2 The Role of the Stirrup Holders

How can less aggressive, ruthless narcissism and more normal, healthy narcissism come into play in the power play in the political arena? It is not possible to distinguish between the good and the evil ruler. It makes no sense to make a division into good and evil, healthy and sick, reasonable, morally impeccable, incorruptible people and pathological narcissistic powerful people corrupted by power. Rather, I would like to give an example:

▶ Example

"The Last King of Scotland—In the Grips of Power" is a 2006 film based on the novel of the same name by Giles Foden (2001). The plot is fictional, but based on events during the reign of Ugandan dictator Idi Amin. The story: The young doctor Nicholas Garrigan *accidentally* meets the new ruler Idi Amin, who calls himself King of Scotland, whom he treats. The latter then convinces him to become his personal physician. Idi Amin is portrayed as an extremely power-mad, narcissistic, megalomaniac and cruel ruler. The young doctor is chosen and favored by the dictator. Only gradually does he become aware of Uganda's horrific history. Although increasingly repulsed by the dictator's atrocities, he succumbs—incomprehensibly for himself—to his charm and charisma. He tries to free himself, but the viewer experiences him as strangely will-less. As a viewer, one understands that he wants to break away from Idi Amin's extremely immoral actions and escape, especially since he is by now certain that he, too, will eventually be killed by Amin. Contrary to this conscious decision, the viewer witnesses Garrigan become will-less as soon as the dictator needs and even abuses him again. He is unable to escape in time and remains in the country. When it is actually already no longer possible, he manages to escape by lucky coincidences and with many losses. As a broken man he returns to his homeland. ◀

Nicholas Garrigan can be seen as a prototype of a narcissistic self-object of a person in power. Giles Foden (2001) has portrayed a character in a novel that can help us understand and possibly avoid incomprehensible and calamitous mistakes that occur in our reality. The reality is that democratic governments repeatedly enter into political friendships with dictators and hold on to them for a long time, until it finally becomes clear that these dictators commit horrendous crimes, grossly violate human rights and are ultimately enemies of every democracy. What is happening cannot be explained on the basis of rational considerations alone.

A political psychoanalysis could reveal in time who is worthy of trust (Wirth 2002), because moral-ethical concerns and benefit-harm analyses alone are not enough (for the economic field, see also Tuckett 2011). A political psychoanalysis could reveal when politicians, mediators and voters of a democratic country have become secondary narcissistic objects of those in power. On their own, they cannot get out of the relational trap of power any more than the protagonist Nicholas Garrigan (Foden 2001). The following problems must be clearly grasped:

- **Problem 1**

Charm and power of seduction on the part of the person in power and seductibility on the part of the victim(s).

- **Problem 2**

Only the failure of the ruler opens the eyes of outsiders to what could previously remain well hidden in the psychosocial arrangement of power.

- **Problem 3**

Those caught in the net could see the immorality and contempt but could not free themselves.

- **Problem 4**

With the impending doom, everyone increasingly understands or feels the ominous downside, namely that an unimaginable destructive and self-destructive potential is released with the offended narcissism and the feared or real loss of power, i.e. powerlessness.

- **Problem 5**

A need for recognition, career ambition, self-centeredness, and thoughtlessness are often seen by the public as signs of leadership strength. There seems to be a fine line between being a strong leader and having violent delusions of grandeur, so the delusion can be overlooked for a time.

- **Problem 6**

Immature personalities, paranoids and psychopaths have a good chance of coming to power or staying in power in dictatorships and monarchies. But who can stop pathological narcissists in a democracy? Presumably the slowness of legislation, the long march through the institutions, the implementing regulations that first have to be enacted, do not succeed in rendering the power-mad person harmless, but they do succeed in limiting him.

- **Problem 7**

It will probably not be possible to keep people with narcissistic personality disorder away from power, because power is sought—as already mentioned—to compensate for feelings of powerlessness, helplessness and inferiority, and therefore exerts an irresistible attraction.

- **Problem 8**

But if the whole responsibility for the phenomena of corrupting and corrupted power is attributed to the powerful, then one sees the errors and causes of the problem only in the other. Then one feels powerless and at the same time finds oneself in a cynical and self-righteous attitude. Then one would have landed in the group of co- or complementary narcissists who hold the stirrups for the narcissist.

When we are dealing with power, we need to keep our own narcissism in mind: What exerts attraction? When are we in danger of falling into a complementary narcissistic stance? Where do our empathic powers fail? Where have we allowed ourselves to be seduced? Where are we corruptible? Where are we willing to be strategic? When do we call ourselves narcissistically healthy and when diseased?

In the therapeutic everyday life we are always searching for a balance in the best case.

8.3 Altruists or Highest Performers?: Cross Your Heart

To ask again with the example in ► Chap. 1, “Are you now more attracted to the people of the altruists or to the people of the highest performers?” Surely almost everyone answers, “To both!”. And it probably depends on the area of the system in which one works, whether in the care of patients, the training of psychotherapists, professional politics, to what extent one lives at times in one people and at other times in the other. In each field of practice, a different mix of professional and personal relationship makes sense. And maybe we just choose the field as our main field of activity, which suits us best.

With regard to daily practice, for which this book was written, it can be stated that we would not get far in daily therapeutic work with a strategy of credibility, persuasiveness and success orientation with full use of our knowledge and skills alone. Patients seek and need genuine relationships in which compassion is extended to them. And many treatment approaches encourage us to bring genuineness and authenticity to encounters and relationships. In this respect, we realize openness and honesty on a very personal level in the therapeutic relationship, which nevertheless also has its very own rules and laws. We must constantly balance an adequate mixture of professional and personal attention to the patient. And patients also have to limit their personal feelings to the area of the professional encounter. However: we can, at least theoretically and in the imagination of patients, more easily withdraw from the relationship, while the patient sees himself in a dependency that can vary in intensity depending on the phase of therapy. It is a fact that once a bond has been formed with a therapist, it is not possible to easily replace him or her. This creates an asymmetry in the relationship. Conscious and unconscious feelings of inferiority, which inevitably arise to a greater or lesser extent as a result, need to be considered, and how they are compensated for. We can, as psychotherapists, work to ensure that the people over whom we have influence (these include ourselves) compensate well for inevitably arising feelings of inferiority and keep their (and we our) narcissistic needs within a healthy range. According to Adler, good, desirable compensation consists in a reduction of vertical structures in favor of the development of compassion and a sense of community and belonging (◘ Fig. 8.1).

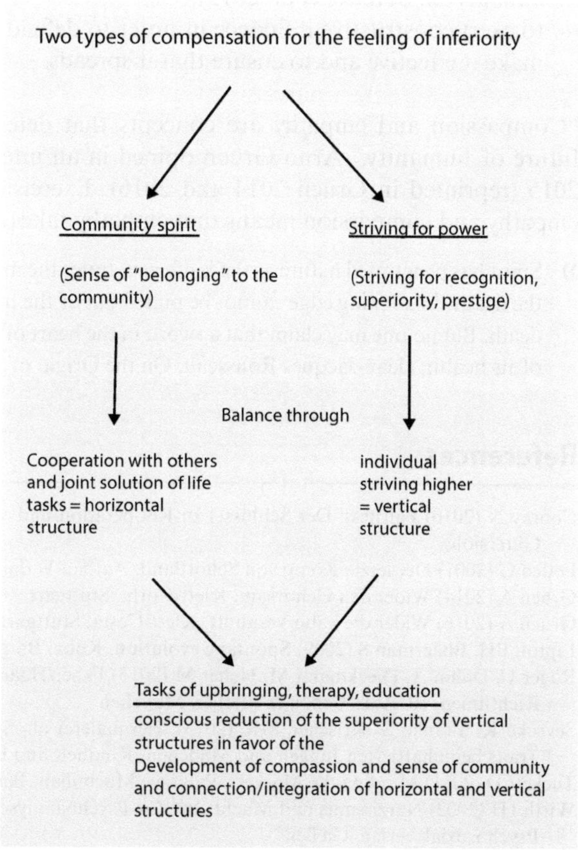

◘ Fig. 8.1 Types of compensation for the feeling of inferiority. (According to Adler)

This compensation is of far-reaching and at the same time also highly political importance, because empathy, feeling with others, as well as the sense of community and belonging form the basis of human coexistence. This basis is still attainable in most people. Therefore, those who can grasp the meaning of compassion and cognitive as well as emotional empathy should be able to feel pain,

- can live and show this openly in a wise way,
- can talk openly about it in appropriate places,
- promote the conversation about it,
- try to learn from our current crises (economy, terror, politics),
- recognize the competitive and profit motive in its effects,
- know what it means that an estimated one third of human beings had an inhuman to cruel childhood, namely that some of them are the most successful of all under conditions of competition and profit precisely because of it,
- recognize when there is a danger of becoming a stirrup holder,
- know that to be able to experience one's own pain and that of the victims is the beginning of change or recovery,
- try to teach others compassion and empathy towards living beings,
- e.g. accelerate the development of relationships characterized by love, compassion and kindness by promoting healthy relationships between children and animals (cf. Sevecke et al. 2013),
- to exert constructive influence in order to defend the power of compassion, to make it effective and to ensure that it spreads.

"Compassion and empathy are concepts that determine the debates about the future of humanity," Arno Gruen opined in an interview on 3Sat on August 30, 2015 (reprinted in Gruen 2014 and 2016). Exercising power and influence with empathy and compassion means that empathy takes on a political dimension.

> Spirit has penetrated nature as the knife penetrates the marrow of a tree. Now, of course, the death-threatening edge cannot be pulled out of the trunk, for the tree would bleed to death. But no one may claim that a sword in the heart of the world's ash tree is the mark of its health. (Jean-Jacques Rousseau, On the Origin of Inequality among Men, 1750)

References

Copray N (2010) Fairness. Der Schlüssel zu Kooperation und Vertrauen. Gütersloher Verlagshaus, Gütersloh

Foden G (2001) Der letzte König von Schottland. Aufbau Verlag, Berlin

Gruen A (2014) Wider den Gehorsam. Klett-Cotta, Stuttgart

Gruen A (2016) Wider die kalte Vernunft. Klett-Cotta, Stuttgart

Lipton BH, Bhaerman S (2009) Spontane evolution. Koha, Burgrain

Rüger U, Dahm A, Dieckmann M, Neher M (2015) Faber/Haarstrick. Kommentar Psychotherapie-Richtlinien, 10. Aufl. Urban & Fischer, München

Sevecke K, Franke S, Krischer MK (2013) Tierquälerei als Symptom von Callous-Unemotional Traits bei inhaftierten Jungen und Mädchen. Kindheit und Entwicklung 22(3):165–173

Tuckett D (2011) Minding the Markets. Palgrave Macmillan, Basingstoke

Wirth HJ (2002) Narzissmus und Macht. In: Zur Psychoanalyse seelischer Störungen in der Politik. Psychosozial-Verlag, Gießen

Supplementary Information

M.-L. Althoff, *Mentalizing Power and Powerlessness*,
https://doi.org/10.1007/978-3-662-66119-2

References

Adler A (1927) Menschenkenntnis. Menschenkenntnis. Fischer, Frankfurt a.M.. 1966

Albani C, Blaser G, Geyer M, Kächele H (1999) Die "Control-Mastery" Theorie – eine kognitiv orientierte psychoanalytische Behandlungstheorie von Joseph Weiss. Forum Psychoanal 15:224–236

Allen JG, Fonagy P (2006) Mentalisierungsgestützte Therapie. Klett-Cotta, Stuttgart. 2009

Allen JG, Fonagy P, Bateman AW (2011) Mentalisieren in der psychotherapeutischen Praxis. Klett-Cotta, Stuttgart. 2008

Althoff ML (2009) Der Sichere Rahmen. Peter Lang, Frankfurt a.M.

Althoff ML (2013) Die vakante Sitzung in Psychoanalyse und Supervision. Forum Psychoanal 29: 139–160

AN (1994) Affect regulation and the origin of the self. Lawrence Erlbaum, Hillsdale, NJ

Arendt H (1963a) Wahrheit und Politik. In: Wahrheit und Lüge in der Politik. Zwei Essays. Piper, München 1972

Arendt H (1963b) Eichmann in Jerusalem. Ein Bericht von der Banalität des Bösen. Piper, München 2011

Bandura A (1976) Lernen am Modell. Ansätze zu einer sozial-kognitiven Lerntheorie. Klett, Stuttgart

Bandura A (1979) Sozial-kognitive Lerntheorie. Klett-Cotta, Stuttgart

Bateman AW, Fonagy P (2006) Psychotherapie der Borderline-Persönlichkeitsstörung. Ein mentalisierungsgestütztes Behandlungskonzept. Psychosozial-Verlag, Gießen. 2008

Bateman AW, Fonagy P (2008) Comorbid antisocial and borderline personality disorder and comorbid antisocial personality disorder: mentalization based treatment. J Clin Psychol 64:1–14

Bateson G (1996) Ökologie des Geistes: anthropologische, psychologische, biologische und epistemologische Perspektiven. Suhrkamp, Frankfurt a.M.

Bauers J (2007) Prinzip Menschlichkeit. Warum wir von Natur aus kooperieren. Hoffmann und Campe, Hamburg

Bergmann-Mausfeld G (2006) Pathologische Passung, Mentalisierung und negative therapeutische Reaktion. Forum Psychoanal 22:249–267

Bergmann-Mausfeld G (2013) Die Vertreibung aus der Hölle. Zur Bindungskraft früher pathogener Bindungserfahrungen. Forum Psychoanal 29:459–475

Bion WR (1959) Angriffe auf Verbindungen. In: Bott Spillius E (Hrsg) (1990) Melanie Klein heute, Bd 1. Verlag Internationale Psychoanalyse, München, S. 110–139

Bischof-Köhler D (2011) Soziale Entwicklung in Kindheit und Jugend – Bindung, Empathie, Theory of Mind. Kohlhammer, Stuttgart

Blair RJR (2005) Responding to the emotions of others: dissociating forms of empathy through the study of typical and psychiatric populations. Conscious Cognit 14:698–718

Böllinger L (2008) Macht. In: Mertens W, Waldvogel B (eds) Handbuch psychoanalytischer Grundbegriffe. Kohlhammer, Stuttgart, pp 441–446

Brandl Y, Bruns G, Gerlach A, Hau S, Janssen PL, Kächele H, Leichsenring F, Leuzinger-Bohleber M, Mertens W, Rudolf G, Schlösser AM, Springer A, Stuhr U, Windaus E (2004) Psychoanalytische Therapie. Eine Stellungnahme für die wissenschaftliche Öffentlichkeit und für den Wissenschaftlichen Beirat Psychotherapie. Forum Psychoanal 20:13–125

Buchheim P, Cierpka M (eds) (2000) Macht und Abhängigkeit. Lindauer Texte. Springer, Berlin Heidelberg

Campbell J (1994) Die Kraft der Mythen. Artemis & Winkler, Zürich

Copray N (2010) Fairness. Der Schlüssel zu Kooperation und Vertrauen. Gütersloh, Gütersloher Verlagshaus

Dreikurs R (2009) Psychologie im Klassenzimmer. Klett-Cotta, Stuttgart

Drewermann E (2005) Dornröschen. Patmos, Ostfildern

Eickelpasch R, Rademacher C (2004) Identität. Transcript Verlag, Bielefeld

Eiguer A (1989) Le pervers narcissique et son complice. Dunod, Paris

Epictet (2004) Handbüchlein der Moral. Reclam, Ditzingen

Ermann M (2005) On perverse thinking. Int Forum Psychoanal 14:188–192

Ferenczi S (1933) Sprachverwirrung zwischen den Erwachsenen und dem Kind. In: Schriften zur Psychoanalyse, Bd 2. Fischer, Frankfurt a.M. 1972
Fink-Eitel H (1992) Dialektik der Macht. In: Angehrn E et al (eds) Dialektischer Negativismus. Suhrkamp, Frankfurt a.M., pp 35–56
Foden G (2001) Der letzte König von Schottland. Aufbau Verlag, Berlin
Fonagy P (2003) Bindungstheorie und Psychoanalyse, 3. Aufl. Klett-Cotta, Stuttgart, p 2009
Fonagy P, Target M (1998) Ein interpersonelles Verständnis des Säuglings. In: Hurry A (Hrsg) (2002) Psychoanalyse und Entwicklungsförderung von Kindern. Brandes & Apsel, Frankfurt a.M., S. 11–42
Fonagy P, Target M (2006) Psychoanalyse und die Psychopathologie der Entwicklung. Klett-Cotta, Stuttgart
Fonagy P, Gergely G, Jurist E, Target M (2004a) Affektregulierung, Mentalisierung und die Entwicklung des Selbst. Klett-Cotta, Stuttgart
Fonagy P, Gergely G, Jurist EL, Target M (2004b) Entwicklungsaufgaben der normalen Adoleszenz und adoleszenter Zusammenbruch. In: Fonagy P, Gergely G, Jurist EL, Target M (eds) Affektregulierung, Mentalisierung und die Entwicklung des Selbst. Klett-Cotta, Stuttgart, pp 320–342
Foucault M (1987) Das Subjekt und die Macht. In: Hubert L, Dreyfus PR (eds) Michel Foucault. Jenseits von Strukturalismus und Hermeneutik. Athenäum, Frankfurt a.M., pp 241–261
Freud S (1915) Bemerkungen über die Übertragungsliebe. GW X, S. 306–321
Freud S (1920) Jenseits des Lustprinzips. GW XIII, S. 1–69
Freud S (1932) Warum Krieg? GW XVI, S. 13–27
Fromm E (1976) Haben oder Sein. Deutsche Verlags-Anstalt, München
Fromm E (1981) Märchen, Mythen, Träume. Rowohlt, Reinbek b. Hamburg
Gergely G, Watson J (1996) Die Theorie des sozialen Biofeedbacks durch mütterliche Affektspiegelung. Selbstpsychologie 17/18:143–194
Gergely G, Watson J (1999) Early social-emotional development: Contingency perception and the social biofeedback model. In: Rachat P (ed) Early social cognition: understanding others in the first months of life. Erlbaum, Hillsdale, NJ, pp 101–137
Gilligan C (1983) Die verlorene Stimme. Campus, Frankfurt a.M.
Goleman D (2008) Soziale Intelligenz. Knaur, München
Greenson R (1967) The technique and practice of psychoanalysis, vol 1. International Universities Press, New York
Grof S (1975) Topographie des Unbewussten: LSD im Dienst der tiefenpsychologischen Forschung. Klett-Cotta, Stuttgart
Gruen A (1984) Der Verrat am Selbst. Die Angst vor Autonomie bei Mann und Frau. Causa, München
Gruen A (2014) Wider den Gehorsam. Klett-Cotta, Stuttgart
Gruen A (2016) Wider die kalte Vernunft. Klett-Cotta, Stuttgart
Gruen A, Weber D (2001) Hass in der Seele. Herder, Freiburg i.B
Habermas J (1981) Philosophisch-politische profile. Suhrkamp, Frankfurt a.M.
Habermas J (1985) Die neue Unübersichtlichkeit. Kleine Politische Schriften V. Suhrkamp, Frankfurt a.M.
Häusel HG (2008) Brain view. Haufe, Planegg
Hesse H (1987) Demian. GW Bd. 5. Suhrkamp, Frankfurt a.M.
Hinsch R, Pfingsten U (2007) Das Gruppentraining sozialer Kompetenzen (GSK). Grundlagen, Durchführung, Materialien. Beltz, Weinheim
Hirigoyen MF (2002) Die Masken der Niedertracht. dtv, München
Hurni M, Stoll G (1999) Der Hass auf die Liebe. Psychosozial-Verlag, Gießen
Hüther G (2006) Die Macht der inneren Bilder. Vandenhoeck & Ruprecht, Göttingen
Janov A (1981) Gefangen im Schmerz. Fischer, Frankfurt a.M.
Janov A (1993) Der neue Urschrei: Fortschritt in der Primärtherapie. Fischer, Frankfurt a.M.
Janov A (2000) The biology of love. Prometheus, New York
Janov A (2007) Die Janov-Lösung. Primärtherapie – Ein Weg aus der Depression. SterlinHouse Books, Pittsburgh
Jurist EL (2008) Mind and yours. In: Jurist EL, Slade A, Bergner S (eds) Mind to mind. Infant research, neuroscience and psychoanalysis. Other Press, New York

Kahl-Popp J (2010) Kontextanalytische Supervision in der psychoanalytischen Ausbildung. Psychotherapeut 55:471–476

Kämmerer A, Funke J (2004) Seelenlandschaften. Streifzüge durch die Psychologie. 98 persönliche Positionen. Vandenhoeck & Ruprecht, Göttingen

Kast V (1983) Mann und Frau im Märchen. Eine psychologische Deutung. Walter, Olten

Kast V (1984) Familienkonflikte im Märchen. Eine psychologische Deutung. Walter, Olten

Kast V (1988) Imagination als Raum der Freiheit. Walter, Olten

Kernberg OF, Dulz B, Eckert J (2005) WIR: Psychotherapeuten über sich und ihren "unmöglichen" Beruf. Schattauer, Stuttgart

Kohlberg L (1974) Zur kognitiven Entwicklung des Kindes. Suhrkamp, Baden-Baden

König K (2008) Brüder und Schwestern. Geburtenfolge als Schicksal, 14. Aufl. Vandenhoeck & Ruprecht, Göttingen

Konrad K, Firk C, Uhlhaas PJ (2013) Hirnentwicklung in der Adoleszenz. Dtsch Ärzteblatt 25:425–431

Kraus B (2002) Konstruktivismus—Kommunikation—Soziale Arbeit. Radikalkonstruktivistische Betrachtungen zu den Bedingungen des sozialpädagogischen Interaktionsverhältnisses. Carl-Auer-Systeme, Heidelberg

Kraus B (2013) Erkennen und entscheiden. Beltz, Weinheim/Basel

Kuiper PC (1980) Die seelischen Krankheiten des Menschen. Huber, Stuttgart

Künkel F (1929) Die Arbeit am Charakter. Die neuere Psychotherapie in ihrer Anwendung auf Erziehung. Selbsterziehung und Seelenführung, Bahn, Schwerin

Künkel F (1935) Grundzüge der praktischen Seelenheilkunde. Hippokrates, Stuttgart

Langs RJ (1982) Psychotherapy: a basic text. Jason Aronson, New York

Langs RJ (1984) Die Angst vor validen Deutungen und vor einem festen Rahmen. Forum Psychoanal 5: 1–18 (1989). Original: Making interpretations and securing the frame. Int J Psychoanal 10:3–23

Langs RJ (1996) The evolution of the emotion-processing mind. With an introduction to mental Darwinism. London, Karnac Books

Langs RJ (2004) Fundamentals of adaptive psychotherapy and counselling. Palgrave, New York

Leman K (2004) Geschwisterkonstellationen – die Familie bestimmt ihr Leben, 6. Aufl. Moderne Verlagsgesellschaft, Frankfurt a.M.

Leuzinger-Bohleber M (2001) Katamnesen – ihre klinische Relevanz. In: Stuhr U, Leuzinger-Bohleber M, Beutel M (eds) Langzeit-Psychotherapie. Perspektiven für Therapeuten und Wissenschaftler. Kohlhammer, Stuttgart

Lipton BH, Bhaerman S (2009) Spontane evolution. Koha, Burgrain

Luhmann N (1975) Macht, 4. Aufl. UTB, Stuttgart 2012

Luyten P, Fonagy P, Lowyck B, Vermote R (2011) Assessment of mentalization. In: Bateman AW, Fonagy P (eds) Handbook of mentalizing in mental health practice. American Psychiatric Pub, Washington, DC, pp 43–65

Machiavelli N (1513) Il Principe. Übs. und hrsg. von Rudolf Zorn. Kröner, Stuttgart. 1972

Meyer AE, Richter R, Grawe K, von der Schulenburg J-M, Schulte B (1991) Forschungsgutachten zu Fragen eines Psychotherapeutengesetzes. Bundesgesundheitsministerium, Bonn

Miller A (1979) Das Drama des begabten Kindes. Suhrkamp, Berlin

Miller A (2007) Dein gerettetes Leben. Suhrkamp, Berlin

Moeller ML (1982) Sich selbst überleben. Kursbuch 70:71–99

Nietzsche F (1874) Unzeitgemäße Betrachtungen – Schopenhauer als Erzieher. Insel, Berlin 1981

Nietzsche F (1980) Sämtliche Werke. Kritische Studienausgabe in 15 Bänden, 3. Aufl. Hrsg. von Giorgio Colli und Mazzino Montinari. dtv, München 2009

Overbeck G (1997) Der Koryphäenkiller. Suhrkamp, Frankfurt a.M.

Panksepp J (2003) Feeling the pain of social loss. Science 302:237–239

Person ES (2003) Feeling strong. How power issues affect our ability to direct our own lives. Harper Collins, London

Piegler T (2003) Macht, Ohnmacht und Machtmissbrauch in psychotherapeutischen Beziehungen. Psychotherapie Forum 3:106–112

Portele G (1989) Autonomie, Macht, Liebe. Konsequenzen der Selbstreferentialität. Suhrkamp, Frankfurt a.M.

Portele G, Roessler K (1994) Macht und Psychotherapie. Ein Dialog. Edition Humanistische Psychologie, Köln
Pross C (2009) Verletzte Helfer. Klett-Cotta, Stuttgart
Rank O (1924) Das Trauma der Geburt und seine Bedeutung für die Psychoanalyse. Psychosozial-Verlag, Gießen. 2007
Reddemann L (2001) Imagination als heilsame Kraft. Klett-Cotta, Stuttgart
Reddy V (2008) How infants know minds. Harvard University Press, London
Riemann F (1961) Grundformen der Angst. Ernst-Reinhardt-Verlag, München
Roth G, Strüber N (2014) Wie das Gehirn die Seele macht. Klett-Cotta, Stuttgart
Rousseau J-J (1750) Über den Ursprung der Ungleichheit unter den Menschen, vol 1995. Felix Meiner, Hamburg
Rüger U, Dahm A, Dieckmann M, Neher M (2015) Faber/Haarstrick. Kommentar Psychotherapie-Richtlinien, 10. Aufl. Urban & Fischer, München
Sandler J (1976) Gegenübertragung und Bereitschaft zur Rollenübernahme. Psyche 30(4):297–305
Sapute AB, Lieberman MD (2006) Integrating automatic and controlled processes into neurocognitive models of social cognition. Brain Res 1079(1):86–97
Schmidbauer W (1977) Die hilflosen Helfer. Über die seelische Problematik der helfenden Berufe. Rowohlt, Reinbek bei Hamburg
Schmidbauer W (1997) Wenn Helfer Fehler machen. Rowohlt, Reinbek bei Hamburg
Schmidbauer W (2011) Das kalte Herz. Von der Macht des Geldes und dem Verlust der Gefühle. Murmann, Hamburg
Schmidbauer W (2015) Kann eine (Lehr-)Analyse ungültig sein? Forum Psychoanal 31:53–68
Schultz-Venrath U (2013) Lehrbuch Mentalisieren. Klett-Cotta, Stuttgart
Sevecke K, Franke S, Krischer MK (2013) Tierquälerei als Symptom von Callous-Unemotional Traits bei inhaftierten Jungen und Mädchen. Kindheit und Entwicklung 22(3):165–173
Simmel G (1900) Philosophie des Geldes. Anaconda, Köln 2009
Smith DL (1991) Hidden conversations. Routledge, London
Sohni H (2011) Geschwisterdynamik. Psychosozial-Verlag, Gießen
Sowarka B (1995) Soziale Intelligenz und soziale Kompetenz. In: Sarges W (ed) Management-Diagnostik. Hogrefe, Göttingen, pp 365–382
Spangenberg E (2014) Behutsame trauma-integration (TRIMB). Klett-Cotta, Stuttgart
Springer A, Gerlach A, Schlösser A-M (eds) (2005) Macht und Ohnmacht. Psychosozial-Verlag, Gießen
Steinbeis N, Bernhardt BC, Singer T (2012) Impulse control and underlying functions of the left DLPFC mediate age-related and age-independent individual differences in strategic social behavior. Neuron 73(5):1040–1051
Sterba R (1934) The fate of the ego in psychoanalytic therapy. Int J Psychoanalysis 15:117–112
Stern D et al (2012) Veränderungsprozesse. Psychosozial-Verlag, Gießen
Taubner S (2008) Entsteht Einsicht im Täter-Opfer-Ausgleich? Eine empirische Studie am Beispiel adoleszenter Gewaltstraftäter. Monatszeitschrift für Kriminologie 91(4):281–294
Taubner S (2015) Konzept Mentalisieren. Psychosozial-Verlag, Gießen
Taubner S, Sevecke K, Nolte T, Roussow T, Bateman AW (2015) Manual for Menalization-based-treatment for conduct-disorder (MBT-CD). Unveröff, Manuskript
Thorwart J (2015) Zur Prävention von Grenzverletzungen in der psychoanalytischen Ausbildung. Forum Psychoanal 31:35–51
Tibone G, Schmieder-Dembek B (2015) Abstinenz und Abstinenzverletzungen in der psychoanalytischen Ausbildung. Forum Psychoanal 31:17–34
Tuckett D (2011) Minding the Markets. Palgrave Macmillan, Basingstoke
Upledger JE (1996) Auf den inneren Arzt hören. Hugendubel, München
Wampold BE (2001) The great psychotherapy debate: Model, methods, and findings. Lawrence Erlbaum Associates, New York
Watzlawick P (1983) Anleitung zum Unglücklichsein. Piper, München
Weber M (1922) Wirtschaft und Gesellschaft. Siebeck, Tübingen
Weiss J (1993) How Psychotherapy Works. Guilford Press, New York
Wiegand-Grefe S, Schuhmacher M (2006) Strukturelle Gewalt in der psychoanalytischen Ausbildung. Psychosozial-Verlag, Gießen

Willi J (1975) Die Zweierbeziehung. Spannungsursachen, Störungsmuster, Klärungsprozesse, Lösungsmodelle. Rowohlt, Reinbek bei Hamburg

Winnicott DW (1965) Reifungsprozesse und fördernde Umwelt. Studien zur Theorie der emotionalen Entwicklung. Psychosozial-Verlag, Gießen. 2002

Wirth HJ (2002) Narzissmus und Macht. Zur Psychoanalyse seelischer Störungen in der Politik. Psychosozial-Verlag, Gießen

Zimbardo PH (2007) Der Luzifer-Effekt. Spektrum-Verlag, Heidelberg. 2008

Internet Addresses

Anonymous (n.d.). www.staufenbiel.ch/bewerbung-karriere/soft-skills/die-wichtigsten-soft-skills/fuehrung.html. (Zuletzt gesehen: 28.02.2016)

Deutsches Institut für Psychotraumatologie (2016) Sexuelle Übergriffe in Psychotherapie, Psychiatrie, und psychologischer Beratung. http://www.psychotraumatologie.de/missbrauch/informationen. (Zuletzt gesehen: 16.03.2016)

Stangl W (2001) Der Begriff der sozialen Kompetenz in der psychologischen Literatur (Version 2.0). p@psych e-zine 3. Jg. http://paedpsych.jk.uni-linz.ac.at/PAEDPSYCH/SOZIALEKOMPETENZ/. (Zuletzt gesehen: 28.02.2016)

GPSR Compliance

The European Union's (EU) General Product Safety Regulation (GPSR) is a set of rules that requires consumer products to be safe and our obligations to ensure this.

If you have any concerns about our products, you can contact us on ProductSafety@springernature.com

In case Publisher is established outside the EU, the EU authorized representative is:

Springer Nature Customer Service Center GmbH
Europaplatz 3
69115 Heidelberg, Germany

Batch number: 10732090

Printed by Printforce, the Netherlands